The True Story of a Fisherman's

Search for Truth

Glenn F. Gately

All italics in Bible quotations denote my emphasis.

ISBN: 9798648328068

Second edition
May 2020

Cover photo: Glenn fishing the Elwha River with his lab Jake in 1978.

Dedication

This book is dedicated to all those searching for truth
and to
Jesus who is the Way, the Truth, and the Life.

Acknowledgements

I thank all the people who helped me write this book. There were a lot. Special thanks to Heather Reseck for doing her best in teaching me how to write and for doing the lion's share of the editing. And special thanks to Luke Droeger for using his AutoCAD skills in drawing the prophetic time line and sanctuary layout.

Preface

In life we have the opportunity to make many choices—in some countries more than others. In the United States where I live, we are blessed with much freedom. We are free to choose where we will live, who we will marry, what kind of car to buy, and who, when, and how to worship, or not to worship at all. But there is one thing that no one is able to choose. We are not able to choose our parents and the belief system we are raised in.

In this world there are many belief systems. To begin with, there is the atheistic belief that there is no God. We are here by chance, by a random occurrence of atoms coming together to form life; and through a long process, that initial life evolves into human beings.

The alternative to this system is that we were created. Most of the religious systems of the world adhere to the existence of a Creator God. However, the beliefs about this Creator God vary widely. Logic tells us that all belief systems cannot be true. *But what is true?*

This book is my life's story and what I found to be true. To learn what I found, you will need to read the rest of this book. But I will share one thing with you now. God loves *you* exceedingly abundantly. He wants you to know that and He wants you to know Him.

God has promised, "You will seek Me and find Me, when you search for Me with all your heart" (Jeremiah 29:13).

Contents

Introduction

From an early age I developed a love for the outdoors and for fishing and hunting. Raised in a Christian home, I attended Christian schools from the second grade to my second year in college. During these years I was taught that if I died before confessing a mortal sin to a priest, I would burn in hell's fire forever. I faithfully attended church and went to confession right up through my time in the Navy and for a while afterward. Then one Sunday, while in church, I realized that what brought me to church each week was the fear of hell's fire. I had heard some graphic sermons about the fire that burns forever, and I did not want to end up there. In spite of my fear of hell, I decided that that was not a good motive for going to church and that day I decided to stop going.

The next ten years of my life were spent doing what I liked best—fishing and hunting. I also went back to school, earning a B.S. in Forestry with a major in Wildlife Management and a M.S. in Zoology with a major in Fisheries, which led to my becoming a fishery biologist with the U.S. Fish and Wildlife Service in Washington State. There I learned how contaminated fish are. I became discouraged as I became more aware about how badly our earth is polluted and I wondered: *Where is this world heading?*

Although I had stopped going to church, I did not stop believing in God, but I do not remember praying that much. In my early years in Christian schools, I must have been taught that Jesus would return some day, but His return was not something I thought about. In college, I took many courses that taught evolution and that people have been living on earth for millions of years. I thought that if our environment is

1

going to get cleaned up, it is up to us to do it. And I did not think that we were up to the task.

It was at this low point in my life that God put it on my heart to look in the Bible for the answer to my question: *Where is this world heading?*

This book is my life's story of how I found God when I was looking for answers about the earth. However, I believe, whether we realize it or not, we are all looking and thirsting for something that will satisfy us, and only knowing our Creator and Redeemer and His overwhelming love for us will truly satisfy our thirst.

The *first part* of this book is the story of my growing up years, sprinkled with some fishing and hunting adventures. The *second part* is the most important. It is about:

- The Bible—the standard of truth
- The science of salvation (how to be saved)
- God's restoration plan
- Why Jesus has not returned 2,000 years after saying, "It is finished!"
- The link between "climate change" and the soon return of Jesus
- Snares of the devil
- The truth about death
- "Foods" that God never put on the food list
- A "healthy" food to be wary of
- Eight principles for a healthy life
- End time messages from three angels
- God's final test of loyalty

Chapter 1
Hooked on Fishing

Simon Peter said to them, "I am going fishing." - John 21:3

My earliest recollection of fishing was on John Henry's Brook. The year was about 1949 when I would have been five years old. My mother would drive my brother and me to a little stream near Hoosick Falls in upstate New York. We always fished from a bridge on a dirt road. The road must have been little traveled as I do not remember having to get out of the way of any cars. The procedure was the same each time. My mother would fill up a pail with water, put a worm on the hook, lower it down and let the current carry it under the bridge. In a very short time, there would be a speckled trout on the hook, and I would reel it in. Before long there would be enough trout in the pail for supper. From that early experience I was hooked on fishing.

Hoosick Falls is where my mother grew up, but when she married my father, New York City became her home and soon it became home for my sister Carol, my brother Chris, and me. My fishing world expanded in the 1950s when my Uncle Lester and Aunt Mae bought property on Lake Champlain. We camped in a tent that first summer and a whole new world of lake fishing opened up to me. The lake was literally a stone's throw from our tent and that summer I was introduced to many kinds of fish.

The following summer my uncle built a camp and we stayed in it. Not long after, my folks bought property next to my uncle's and in 1955 we had our own camp. My mother, a nurse, worked in a blood bank in lower Manhattan. When school was out, she would take the summer off.

My brother Chris and I would help her load the car and we would make the six-hour drive north to the camp.

In front of our camp was Porter's Marsh with acres of bulrushes, lily pads, and submerged aquatic vegetation. The marsh was a nursery area for many kinds of fish. There were openings scattered throughout the marsh where I spent hours fishing. Using my uncle's rowboat, I would sit on the pointed bow causing the stern to rise up, and using an oar half as a paddle and half as a pole, maneuver around the marsh. Here I learned a self-taught paddling style that would one day cause my wife-to-be to jump out of the boat.

I spent as much time observing life in the marsh as I did fishing. There were ducks with their families of ducklings, kingfishers, hawks, muskrats, bull frogs and other wildlife around the marsh. And there were carp, lots of carp. On calm sunny days they would lie motionless near the surface sunning themselves. When one became startled, it would take off like a shot, setting off a chain reaction as it scared other carp, which scared still others until it seemed every carp in the marsh was on the move. One could easily see where they were going by watching the moving bulrushes.

Sometimes I would stretch out on the dock and peer into the water like it was a large aquarium. I saw perch bugs on the submerged vegetation. That's what my uncle called them because we caught yellow perch with them; later I would learn they were dragonfly larvae. One time I observed a young northern pike, the size of a pencil, grab a minnow cross-wise in its mouth, turn it lengthwise, and swallow it.

We had fun catching bowfin. At night, bowfin move toward shore and before dark we would hook on a sunfish or yellow perch for bait and suspend it from a bobber placed a few feet from the dock. We learned from experience it was best to tie our poles to the dock or we would be looking for them out in the lake! In the morning it was a race down to the dock to see what we had caught. Inevitably, the lines would be threaded out through the bulrushes and we would jump into the boat and work our way to the end of the line. Often times the line would be broken or bitten through by the powerful jaws and needle-sharp teeth of the bowfin.

Sometimes we had our lines go from the water clear up to the camp; we put bells on the lines to alert us when a fish was on. Later I built an advanced alarm system in a cigar box consisting of a battery-operated buzzer and lights. When the alarm sounded in the middle of the night, off we would go, flashlights in hand, to see what we had caught. Nine times out of ten, it was a bowfin. Once it was a longnose gar. The locals called them bill fish because a good portion of this barracuda-like fish was mouth, generously filled with teeth, putting even a northern pike to shame.

I was 13 or 14 years old when my folks bought a 14-foot moulded fiber glass boat. It was wide and flat-bottomed. We could sit on the gunnel without it tipping, making it a safe boat for a lake that could get rough with a north or south wind blowing. Powered by a 12-horse Sea King outboard, that boat expanded my horizons. Now I could explore farther up and down the open lake. I learned the good fishing spots like the edges of weed beds and drop offs. Often, I would spend the entire day on the lake, sometimes waiting until I had just enough light to find the entrance into the marsh. I used the silhouettes of trees in the background to guide me in.

One of my favorite places to go for strawberry bass, a name I learned from my uncle for black crappie—isn't strawberry bass much more appealing!—was a duck blind. Hunters usually built a duck blind a couple hundred yards out from Lang's Beach. If the ice did not take the duck blind with it when it went out in the spring, I would tie the boat up to it and catch one strawberry bass after another. The tricky part was keeping the line from tangling in the duck blind.

Spring was the time to fish bullhead. When the ice went out, the water came in and flooded areas normally dry most of the year. Using a gas lantern, we fished at night with hand lines. We kept the line taut by fixing it in a notch cut in the end of a stick stuck in the ground. A bell attached to the line signaled a fish on. Besides bullhead, we usually caught eels, about one eel for every three or four bullhead.

Spring was also the time to "catch" northern pike and chain pickerel, which came into the flooded woods to spawn. From March 15 to May 15 it was legal to shoot or spear these fish on both the New York and

Vermont sides of the lake. Spearing was done from a boat, but shooting was better accomplished from a tree because visibility was better the higher one was from the water. The fish were not actually shot. The concussion from a deer rifle stunned them long enough to scoop them up in a net.

One time my friend Walt and I borrowed an old wooden boat left on shore for such purposes. As we poled the boat along, the back of the boat started coming off and water began rushing in. Guns in hand, we climbed the nearest trees and watched the boat sink. Some other fisherman-hunters rescued us.

One of my favourite fish to catch and eat was walleye. The best time to catch them was around Memorial Day when the wind was from the south. The best place was off the mouth of Putts Creek, which was a 10-minute boat ride from the camp. We fished with a lead-headed jig, baited with half a nightcrawler. The wind would blow the boat along, causing the jig to bounce along the bottom. Walleye are bottom feeders and this put the bait right where they were feeding. Often we would go home with a nice stringer of walleye.

In the summer, we would steer the boat up Putts Creek passing under a railroad trestle to a hole next to a marsh. We usually caught largemouth bass and yellow perch there. On one occasion, my cousin Bill cast out a Rapala, a lure imitating a small fish, and caught a four-pound brown trout. Another time, my friend Jim caught a twelve-inch rainbow trout on a rubber worm.

I spent many hours fishing in Lake Champlain, but my favourite fishing was on a stream. There were plenty of good trout streams within a short drive of the camp. The closest one and the one that I have fished more than any other stream was Putts Creek. On a map you will find it listed as Putnam Creek, but I have never heard anyone refer to it by that name.

Many a day my mother would drop my friends and me off at the Factoryville Bridge and we would fish it downstream to the bridge near the GLF farm store. Putts Creek had brook, brown, and rainbow trout. It was a rare day that I did not have a limit of ten when my mother picked us up.

I fished other more famous Adirondack streams like the Ausable River and Boquet River, but mostly I fished small streams not far from the camp. There was something about fishing a stream and anticipating what was lurking in each new hole around the next bend.

Sherman Lake, located a half-hour drive from the camp, was another favourite fishing place. Frequently, we went there to catch live bait for our lake fishing. We set minnow traps baited with bread, and sometimes used a drop net off the big rock on the shore. There was always a good supply of golden shiners and other minnows. Sherman Lake was also home to some large brook trout, which tend to grow larger in lakes than in streams. The largest brook trout I have ever caught, two and one-half pounds, came from there. To me, brook trout are the prettiest fish, especially in late September when approaching spawning time and their bellies turn a golden colour.

But the best time to fish Sherman Lake was as soon as the ice began to melt and retreat from the shore. One of my fond memories is taking my mother out when most of the lake was still ice-covered and there was still snow in the woods. We warmed some soup on a fire near the shore and caught a nice mess of trout.

My last memory of Sherman Lake is still fresh in my mind. It was on a trip made in October from my home in Washington. I stood on the big rock, and in a panoramic view, took in the scenery. It was a windless, sunny day. The white birch trees lining the shoreline and magnificent fall foliage of maple, oak, beech, birch, and aspen trees reflected on the lake surface—the perfect scene for a post card.

In every season there were fish to catch and winter was no exception. Occasionally, especially on a three-day weekend, we would visit the camp in winter. Usually, there was snow on the private road that led through an apple orchard, over a railroad track, and around a cow pasture, but sometimes it was plowed by the caretaker of the apple orchard.

Winters in Crown Point were cold. I remember reading the record low was 48 degrees below zero. In the early days at the camp there was only one-quarter inch of asbestocite siding separating the outside from the inside. There was only a Sears and Roebuck wood stove for heat and an outdoor outhouse. Later my folks added inside walls with insulation, and a bathroom. However, since the camp's water was pumped from the lake, running water was available only during the summer months, so we used the outhouse during the rest of the year.

In the winter, cutting holes through two to three feet of ice with an iron ice bar was one way to keep warm. My ice bar was hand-crafted by my cousin Bill, who operated a machine and welding shop in Troy. As the holes were cut and skimmed, tip-ups were baited with minnows and placed in the holes. We jigged with a hand line in one of the holes, while we kept an eye on the tip-ups. When a fish took the bait on a tip-up, the flag would go up. The first to see it would holler, "Tip-up!" The fish would take out line from a spool, which was underwater to prevent it from freezing. The fish we caught ice fishing were yellow perch, northern pike, chain pickerel, and walleye.

Smelt were another fish sought after by ice fisherman. Smelt are a forage fish for the larger game fish and winter is the only time fishermen angle for them. Since smelt do not frequent the area of the lake near the camp, we drove north to Port Henry or Westport to fish for them. Like most fishermen I cut two holes side-by-side, and used two jigging sticks with a heavy torpedo-shaped sinker at the bottom of each line, and two snelled-hooks above the sinker. Bait was a silvery slab of skin cut from the side of a smelt. Often I would be fishing deep and needed a heavy sinker to get down fast. Smelt typically run about six inches long and the sinker weighed about as much as the smelt.

Jigging is done with an up and down motion of the sixteen-inch jigging stick. When fishing deep, one needs experience to discern when a smelt is hooked, so as not to waste time bringing up empty hooks. I learned to tell if a smelt was hooked on the downward motion of the jigging stick. Without a fish on, I would feel a sharp tug as the sinker came down sharply. With a fish on, there was no sharp tug. Because smelt run in large schools, I either filled a pail with them or got skunked. Smelt are soft-bodied fish and easy to clean with a pair of shears. Snip off the head, snip open the belly, remove the entrails and you are done. Fried up, they make a tasty meal, bones and all.

Fishing in the winter was much like fishing any other time of the year. Sometimes I got 'em and sometimes I didn't. I remember calendars that forecasted the best times to go fishing. Dots were placed in the days of the month—the larger the dot, the better the fishing. I think the dots were tied to the phases of the moon. I never paid any attention to these calendars. I went by two rules: 1) the best time to go fishing is when you have the time; and 2) you won't catch any fish unless you have a line in the water!

I am thankful for my early childhood summers living at the camp. Lakes, streams, forests, and fields—how different it was from life in the city. I am thankful for a mother who took summers off from work so that my brother and I could enjoy life at the camp. And I am thankful for a father who supported his family by earning a living in the city although it limited his enjoyment of the camp to vacations and weekends.

Chapter 2
Growing Up in New York City

Train up a child in the way he should go, And when he is old he will not depart from it.
- Proverbs 22:6

I started the first grade in Public School 33, which was right around the corner from the five-story apartment building where we lived at 2400 Davidson Avenue in the Bronx.

My mother was raised in the Episcopalian Church but became a Catholic when she married my father. So in the second grade I transferred to the Catholic school, Saint Nicholas of Tolentine, a few blocks away. The Dominican nuns taught me from grades two through eight and then I learned from the Augustinian priests in high school. After graduating from high school, I attended Manhattan College where I was taught by Jesuit brothers.

When I was about eight years old, I had an eye-opening experience about the truthfulness of newspapers. It was the first day of school and a reporter was there to take some pictures. The next day, there in the centerfold was a picture of my brother Chris. There he was peeking in the school door holding an apple behind his back.

The caption read, "Chris Gately is late for school, but he brought an apple for the teacher." Well I knew that Chris was actually very early and he did not bring an apple. The reporter set him up! At a young age, I learned you cannot trust newspapers to tell the truth.

The block I grew up on was a melting pot of different nationalities and religions. There were Italians, Polish, Puerto Ricans, and African-

Americans coming from Catholic, Protestant, and Jewish faiths. I think the majority were Irish Catholic with names like O'Leary, O'Shaughnessy, O'Donnell, Kilkerry, and McSherry. Gately is also Irish. My daughters, Dawn and Heather, visited Ireland a few years ago. They kept an eye out for some Gately's, but did not meet any.

Although there were parks in the neighborhood with "Keep off the Grass" signs, the street was our playground. There we played stickball using a broom handle for a bat and manhole covers and car fenders for bases. Both sides of the street were lined with five-story buildings; hitting the ball onto nearby roof tops constituted an "out," whereas hitting it onto farther roof tops was a "home run."

We also played touch football, and when snow was on the ground, we played ice hockey without skates. At the fire hydrant we played "triangle," hitting a pitched ball with our hand. At the four-way intersection at the end of the block, we played "four corners," hitting the ball on the point of the curb. Storm-water drains on the corners were bases. When the ball went down a drain opening, we fished it out with a modified coat hanger. We played basketball on the sidewalk and shot "baskets" through the rungs of the fire escape ladder. Once in a while, we rode our bikes to Van Courtland Park, which had woods, fields, and a lake. The lake had mostly goldfish and the fishing was not very good.

Fishing Near the City

I did get to do some fishing in the Saw Mill River, about 20 miles away. Trout season opened on April 1 and when the *Daily News* and *Daily Mirror* came out the next day, you could be sure the centerfolds would have pictures of fishermen elbow-to-elbow lining the Saw Mill River. Any trout fisherman worthy of the name knew that this was not the way to catch trout. Trout by nature are a wily fish that spook easily and head for the nearest cover. In spite of this fact, few trout fishermen after a long-closed season could resist the urge to get out. So, my father would take along some reading material and drive me to the stream. Usually I did not catch anything on opening day, but one year I caught a brook trout, just barely meeting the seven-inch size requirement. The word got out and soon fishermen were coming to see my prize fish. I felt really important that day.

A couple times I walked to the Harlem River with my bait casting rod and practiced casting a one-ounce Daredevil at objects floating down the river. I walked out to the end of an old abandoned pier that had nothing left to walk on but twelve-inch wide beams. One miss-step here would send me into the river. Boy was I surprised one day when I turned around to see my mother behind me. I do not know how she knew where I was. Mothers have a way of knowing.

When I was older, I went fishing near Englewood Cliffs on the New Jersey side of the Hudson River. We mostly caught tomcod, but once I reeled in a blue crab. With the crab dangling from my fishing pole, I asked the fellow fishing next to me, "You want this crab?"

"Sure, I'll take it," he responded.

I swung my rod toward him for him to take it off. Before you knew it, the crab latched onto his hand with one of its claws. I went to help him pry it off and while I was helping him, the other claw grabbed his cheek. Now the crab was suspended between his hand and his cheek. He was turning red in the face and tears were welling up in his eyes. He was really hurting. It took all my strength to pry open the pincers and get the crab off him. His cheek never bled, but there were deep indentations left on the side of his face. My fingers were sore for several days afterward.

Other fishing opportunities in the city included party boats that took fishermen out into Long Island Sound. I have experienced three fishing expeditions on party boats, one with my sister, Carol, and two with neighborhood kids from the block. Fishing from a party boat was like fishing the Saw Mill River on opening day. We fished elbow-to-elbow along the side of the boat. We caught flounder, fluke, and porgies on those trips. On my first trip I won the pool with the biggest fish. On my second trip, I came in second. And on my third trip I was out of the running.

On one of those trips I was pulling in fish two at a time when the man fishing next to me was not catching anything. He wanted to know what I was using for bait. I was using sand worms, just like he was. Then he asked me if I would bait his hooks for him, which I did. I can't remember if it helped him or not.

Hunting

Besides fishing, I naturally took to hunting. When I was fourteen years old, I went to the Davega Sporting Goods store on Fordham Road with my father to get my first hunting license. Because of my young age, my father had to sign across the license. My early days of hunting were done near the camp or with my cousin Bill near his home in Troy. Within walking distance of his house there were fields and woods and lots of cottontail rabbits as well as ring-necked pheasants.

I used to like to track pheasants on fresh snow when it snowed during the night. One time I was following tracks that ended. When a pheasant takes off on the snow, it leaves wing marks on both sides of the tracks, but here there were no wing marks. I stood there looking down at the last track wondering what had become of it when I noticed a little hole smaller than a dime and an eye looking up at me. I thought, *I am going to catch a pheasant in my hands!* I put my gun down and slowly moved my hands toward the pheasant. When my hands were about a foot above the snow, the pheasant burst out, showering me with snow. I never have caught a pheasant in my hands.

Another time, I was tracking a rabbit and was looking down following the tracks when right by my feet I spotted a grouse. Quickly, I reached down and grabbed it by the head. That's when I realized it was frozen and must have died during the night. Its feathers were all fluffed up the way birds do when it is cold.

Saved from Harm

In my early days of hunting I used my mother's shotgun, an old Lefever double-barrel twenty-gauge. I am sorry to say that that gun is no more and I am responsible. During my first forty years of life, I did a lot of reloading for both shotgun and rifle. I was in my teens when I first started with a Lee Reloader purchased for nine dollars and ninety-five cents. I learned the hard way that it is not good to deviate from the prescribed measurements of powder and shot. My friend Walt and I were experimenting with different combinations of powder and shot and taking turns shooting. It was Walt's turn shooting with me standing next

13

to him when part of the chamber blew away and the ventilated rib between the barrels took the form of a horseshoe. Looking back, I believe that was one of the times God saved my life and He saved Walt's life too.

In 1962, my father bought a Chevy II, the only car he bought new in his entire life. I got to drive it frequently and would drive it to the camp over the next few years. One day I decided to drive to the camp on the Vermont side of the lake. Young and foolish, I decided to see how fast the Chevy II would go. On a long straightaway, I pressed the accelerator to the floor and watched the speedometer reach 100 miles per hour. It turned out that the long straightaway was not long enough. I could see the road ahead curving to the right and knew the car was not going to slow down in time to make it. Providentially, I saw a logging road straight ahead. I crossed the left lane, entered the logging road, and got the car slowed down and stopped. If the logging road had not been there, it would have crashed into a tree for sure. I believe God, who knows the end from the beginning, had that road put there to save my life.

Starting College

Based on tests taken early in high school, students were placed on one of two paths, commercial or academic. I started on the academic path with the assumption that I would go on to college. But what kind of college should I go to? I was very naïve about the possible choices for a career. I thought there were only three choices: liberal arts, business, and engineering. I always had an interest in electricity, which may have come from playing with Lionel trains and building electric motors. So I chose electrical engineering. In the fall of 1962, I started attending Manhattan College's School of Engineering in the Bronx.

In 1963, in the middle of my third semester, I came home to find my father dead in his chair from a heart attack. He was only fifty-four years old. He had stopped working several years before due to his heart condition. I lost interest in school and withdrew from school without finishing my third semester.

The Great Northeast Blackout

After my father's death I went to work for the Central Foundry Company, which made cast iron pipe fittings for high-rise buildings. I began working at a warehouse in Queens and later was promoted to the main office at 932 Broadway in Manhattan. I commuted to Manhattan on the subway. In November 1965 I experienced the Great Northeast Blackout when the power went off in eight northeast states and Ontario, Canada.

I was on the train between stations when the power went off. After an hour or so of waiting, they opened the doors and we walked by flashlight along the catwalk to the nearest station. It was an eerie feeling coming up out of the subway and seeing New York City in total darkness, except for the headlights of cars.

How was I to get home? I mostly walked since the buses were jam-packed and people were even riding on the bumpers outside. As I headed toward home, I encountered garbage cans on fire, bus doors lying in the street, people breaking into stores, and alarms going off.

When I finally made it home late that night, I had to get my car from a parking building where I had left it the day before because I could not find a parking space. When I got there, there were two people in a booth counting money with a flashlight. I asked if I could use the flashlight to find my car, but they said they needed it. With a little moonlight filtering in through the open sides of the building, I began walking up the spiral driveway trying to figure out when I was on the level where my car was. Amazingly, I found it by feeling cars when I thought I was in the right area. By the next morning the power was back on and life in the city was back to normal.

Chapter 3
Navy Life

A great windstorm arose, and the waves beat into the boat, so that it was already filling. - Mark 4:37

On April 14, 1965 I turned twenty one. At that time the Vietnam War was going strong and the draft was on. My brother Chris had joined the Marines the previous September at the age of 17 and was already in Vietnam. I figured it would not be long before I was drafted, so I decided that if I had to be in the service, I would make my own choice in the matter. Liking the water so much, I decided to join the Navy Reserves in Yonkers, New York.

One week after signing the papers, my draft notice arrived in the mail. It contained a fifteen-cent subway token, my paid transportation to Whitehall Street, where I was to be inducted into the army. I turned the letter over to the Chief at the Naval Reserve Center and he said he would take care of it. I didn't hear any more from the draft board until several months later when I received a letter telling me to return the subway token. In those days a postage stamp was three cents and I never did return it.

USS Bristol DD-857

My first year in the reserves consisted of attending weekly meetings and a two-week training cruise on the destroyer USS Bristol DD-857. I boarded the ship at the Brooklyn Navy Yard in February 1966, and we shoved off for sunny San Juan, Puerto Rico. However, between Brooklyn and San Juan, it was not that sunny.

Somewhere off Cape Hatteras, North Carolina we hit a storm. My berth was in the bow along the skin of the ship. We were doing a lot of rolling from side to side and pitching up and down. I was sleeping with one arm around a pipe to keep from sliding off the rack when someone woke me up and told me I had to get up and help bail the ship out. Being a reservist, I thought this was some kind of hazing. However, as soon as I swung my feet onto the deck and felt cold water, he didn't have to do any more convincing.

I asked, "Where's the bucket?" Soon I was on a bucket line, passing the bucket from one person to the next and dumping it into a shower stall where it drained out. As the ship rolled and pitched it was all we could do to stand up. People were getting sick and throwing up and the bucket line was getting thinner. I ended up being the only one in the head. The buckets were placed just inside the hatchway and I had to carry them to the shower stall. When I could not get to a bucket fast enough and the ship rolled the bucket would fly across the deck hitting me in the shins.

When the storm was over, I saw how the water was coming in. The forward 5-inch gun mount had caved in from the force of the water. When we arrived in San Juan, the weather was calm and sunny and I enjoyed some of the whitest beaches I have ever seen.

Active Duty

A few months later, in May, it was time to start my two years of active duty. The Navy approved my request to attend electronic technician school, which took me to the Great Lakes Naval Training Center in Illinois. After a few days I realized I could fish nearby but I had not brought any fishing gear. I met another sailor, Dan, who wanted to go home to Pittsburg and bring back his car, so I made plans to fly home, get my fishing gear, and meet him in Pittsburgh. Since neither one of us had much money, we could not drive far on the toll roads. When it was my turn to drive, he told me to pump the brakes a lot when I needed to stop. The first red light I saw up ahead I started pumping. I pumped and pumped and sailed right through the red light. Fortunately, there were no cars coming and somehow, we made it back to the Naval

Station.

Fishing and Hunting Again

While in Illinois, I got to do some fishing on the great Mississippi River. I don't remember catching anything, but I was impressed with how wide the river was and what a maze of side channels there were. Each side channel interconnected with another one and you could go quite far from the main channel. It would be easy to get lost in those side channels and it could take a while to find your way out. Fortunately, we made it out.

As the end of training approached, I filled out a "dream sheet" with a request for my next duty station. I put in for a destroyer on the East Coast. I must have forgotten about my experience on the Bristol. Anyway, I did not get it. I was assigned an aircraft carrier, the USS Kitty Hawk CVA 63, out of San Diego. Based on what happened to two guys who graduated with me, I don't think they bothered to even look at the requests. One put in for Norfolk, Virginia and the other for Newport, Rhode Island. Each got what the other requested.

Before reporting for duty, I had some leave time coming, just in time for the October deer season at the camp. My friend Red, a rodeo bull rider from the Bronx, his black lab, and I headed for the camp. In a day or two Red and I drove out on a forest road to Hammond Pond to hunt Burnt Ridges, mountains burned by a fire in the past.

I have a tendency to go up hill when I hunt and before long was in a little saddle between two ridges. It was a nice day with no snow on the ground. I put my back up against a tree and was soon snoozing. I was awakened by rustling leaves as a ruffed grouse walked by. Not long after that came a fork-horn which I shot. After gutting the deer, I started dragging it out. Although it was pretty much a downhill drag, sunset comes early in October and I was running out of daylight. I decided to leave the deer so I could travel faster. I marked the spot and traveled down the mountain, following a dry streambed. Soon the sun was down and the moon was out. I could see Hammond Pond glimmering below me in the moonlight and I made it to the pond and followed the forest road to where the truck was parked. I was ravenous by this time and was looking forward to some food I had left in the truck. When I got there, Red was there but the food wasn't; he had eaten everything. He never heard me shoot and did not believe me that I had shot a deer. We returned the next day, found the deer, and then he believed me.

Before heading back to the Bronx, Red and I decided to hunt crows. Red parked his pickup on the side of the road. We walked up onto a little knoll and positioned ourselves underneath some evergreen trees. I turned on the portable record player I had made and started playing a record of crows in distress. Before any crows came in, the toot of a horn drew our attention to Red's pickup, which we saw slowly rolling backwards. It went off the side of the road and knocked down a few old fence posts. Red's dog had knocked the truck out of gear and gotten our attention by honking the horn as it was rolling. We got the truck back on the road and drove back to the camp. I don't remember shooting any crows.

Heading home the next day, I got to drive Red's pickup. I have never driven a vehicle with so much play in the wheel. By the time we arrived in the Bronx my arms were worn out. We brought the deer into Red's apartment and butchered it. As we were skinning it out with its front legs tied up high, one of them slipped loose and hit me in the forehead right between the eyes. The deer had his revenge!

USS Kitty Hawk CVA 63

Before long I was on my way to Japan to board the Kitty Hawk. As it turned out, the ship was still in San Diego and I could have boarded there, but this gave me some time to see Japan so I did not complain. In about a week, the ship came in and I began life as an electronic technician or ET. There were about one hundred ET's in the division in two shops. Each shop was divided into two twelve-hour shifts, a day shift and a night shift. I was assigned to the day shift in Shop 2. It was no surprise to us that our destination was the South China Sea off Vietnam in an area known as Yankee Station. The war was at the height of the bombing and for twelve hours a day we launched sorties of F-4 Phantoms, A-4 Skyhawks, and A-6 Intruders. Flight ops (operations) were timed so that after one sortie was launched, a returning sortie landed. When we were not having flight ops, I would go out on the catwalk or sit in the nets on the bow and look for flying fish and sea snakes.

The Hawk was not the only carrier on Yankee Station. The Ranger, Constellation, Bonhomie Richard, and Enterprise were also there at times. There were usually three carriers on duty all the time. After about thirty-five days on Yankee Station, we would head to Subic Bay in the Philippines for some R & R. When North Korea captured the USS Pueblo in January 1968 and the Enterprise left Yankee Station for North Korea, we had to fill in and stayed out over sixty days before going to Subic Bay. It seemed like a long time.

At the mouth of Subic Bay was Grande Island. It had concrete bunkers and gun emplacements built during World War II that looked very similar to the ones on Marrowstone Island where I live now. Grande Island had a pier and I got in some fishing there and caught some bonito, a hard fighting fish. All day long on Grande Island there were steaks on the grill and soda to drink at no charge. For recreation, there was a miniature golf course and a swimming pool. Due to my near-sightedness, I mistakenly dove in at the shallow end. My head hit the concrete bottom and things became foggy as I walked out of the pool with blood streaming down my face. I thought about going back to the ship on the next liberty launch for some first aid, but did not. I put my blue work cap on and the bleeding stopped. In a few days the cut healed and my recovery was complete.

The other alternative for taking liberty in Subic Bay was going to Olongapo, the nearest town. Most of Olongapo was off limits except for the main street which consisted of one bar after another. I have to admit I tried them out, but most of the time I headed for Grande Island. We had to be careful about wearing a wristwatch in Olongapo. Expert watch thieves could get them off your wrist in a flash as you walked down the street. Then the thief or his accomplice would make the rounds through the bars with a tray of watches for sale, giving us the opportunity to buy the watch back or upgrade to a better one.

On one of the Hawk's trips to Subic Bay a few of us took leave and went to Baguio City, a mountain resort at a cool and refreshing 5,000 feet elevation. On the way there, the young Philippine men traveling with us showed us their skill in opening beer bottles with their teeth. As we neared Baguio, I was greeted with the familiar scent of pine trees, reminding me of the camp. It cooled down at night and we built a fire in the fireplace. We bought pizza but had to fry it because what we thought was an oven below the stove burners turned out to be a refrigerator.

I liked using my training to repair the equipment I was responsible for. Mostly I worked on UHF and VHF transmitters and receivers, but once in a while on radar repeaters. Although transistors were used in the aircraft's radios in the 1960s, most of the ship's gear used vacuum tubes. This made it possible to find the faulty component on a printed circuit board and replace it. Today with integrated circuits, the entire circuit board would be replaced—not nearly as challenging.

I also worked on a bank of RCTU's (Remote Control Telephone Units). These were an interface between a transmitter/receiver and a hand set. From the time I got on board, one of the units could not be used because of a short. Because there were extra units, this faulty one was ignored. Liking a challenge, I gathered blueprints of where the cable went on the ship and when we were in port I started narrowing down the location of the short. The search led me to parts of the ship I would have never seen. In one compartment I removed a metal cover plate from the bulkhead covering a terminal board. As soon as the plate came off I saw a wire that had been pinched between the bulkhead and cover plate. I thought to myself, *I bet that this is the shorted wire,* and it was. Now all the RCTU's were working.

I made two cruises to Vietnam within my two-year obligation. Although part of the war, we never got close enough to Vietnam to see land and I never feared for my safety unlike my brother Chris, who saw combat and was wounded on December 21, 1965. I vividly remember my mother answering the doorbell in the middle of the night to receive the telegram from Western Union. Although bad news, we were thankful it was not the worst news that some 60,000 other mothers received during the war. The war was very real to our pilots, some returning with holes in their planes and some not returning at all.

Chapter 4

Discharged

Now the LORD had said to Abram: "Get out of your country, from your family and from your father's house, to a land that I will show you." -
Genesis 12:1

In May 1968, I was discharged from the navy and went home to New York. Before looking for work, I decided to take the summer off and do some camping. I found a 1957 Volkswagen microbus that had been converted into a camper. It had a lot of rust as most cars do after driving on New York's salted roads, but my cousin Bill patched it up and even gave it a coat of green paint. I loaded up my fishing gear, sleeping bag, and other essentials and headed north for Canada to catch some big ones. The camper proved to be comfortable. The chair at the table folded into a bed and I used cans of Sterno to cook hot meals.

Lost in the Woods

Before long I was in Quebec's La Verendrye Park heading east on Penetration Road, a ninety-five-mile dead end road. I had no particular destination in mind; I was just looking for a place to fish. I crossed a river and then came to a small stream that looked inviting. I parked the bus, got out my fishing pole and headed into the woods. When I started, it was cool and there were no biting insects around, but as it warmed up the black flies came out in force. The stream flowed through a lot of tag alders and I made a little circle to get around a particularly thick bunch. I kept circling and circling, but could not find the stream! By this time the black flies were really making a meal out of me and I had to keep moving to get any respite, but the tag alders were so thick that I could not move fast enough to get away from them. To move faster, I took the reel off my fishing pole and stuck the pole in the ground.

Eventually, I found the stream, but by this time I could not be sure it was the same one I started on! Whether it was or not, I figured it had to empty into the river I had driven past and decided to follow it downstream to the river and then follow the river back to Penetration Road. I was feeling a little lost and did not want to get *really* lost. According to my road map there was nothing but a railroad track between me and Hudson Bay. I knew I was on the north side of Penetration Road, but did not have a compass with me and the sun was not out to guide me. After a while it started getting dark and I resigned myself to spend the night in the woods. One good thing is that black flies go to bed when it gets dark. I built a little fire and cooked the one small brook trout I had caught. I was so hungry I ate everything there was to eat on that fish.

After that small supper, I put my back against a tree and started dozing. *WHAM!* I jumped! A beaver had slapped the water with its tail only a few feet away. In the morning I was glad to see the sun come up. I revised my plan, used the sun to get my bearings, and headed south. In a little while I came out to Penetration Road. The land I came out over was rather steep—totally different from the flat land I went in on. I was not entirely sure which way to walk on Penetration Road, but guessed right and after a half hour's walk was greeted by the sight of my green VW bus. I learned on this trip north that the fish in Canada were no bigger than what I was used to catching in New York. I also learned to always take insect repellent, matches, and a compass with me when going into a remote area.

Bugle

I spent the rest of the summer at the camp and enjoyed fishing in the lake and trout streams. I bought a hunting dog from my farmer friend who owned the mother, a black and tan coon hound, whose name was Music, but we called her Musey. The father was a bluetick hound. I named my dog Bugle and at eight weeks I started training him on rabbits. I would shoot a rabbit, drag it along the ground, and then let Bugle smell his way to it.

Hounds are not noted for retrieving, but when he was a few months older I gave it a try. I threw a ball out and Bugle ran out to get it and brought it right back to me. I threw it out again and Bugle did the same thing. The third time I threw it out, he walked out to it, lifted his leg, peed on the ball, and walked away. After that if I picked up the ball, Bugle would yawn and walk into his doghouse. I did nothing for a while after that until I saw him pick up the ball one day. I threw it out and he brought it back. This time I did not press it. But once in a while, when it had cooled down in the evening, I would throw it once or twice, but never more than that. That little training paid off.

When hunting season opened that fall, whether I shot a rabbit, squirrel, or grouse, Bugle brought it back to me. He also hunted raccoon at night, and if there were any low limbs in the tree the coon was in, Bugle was up the tree as high as he could go. There was never any doubt which tree the coon was in.

One time my friend Andy was at the camp with his black lab Jud, an experienced duck retriever. We had a retrieving contest between Bugle and Jud. We lined the two dogs up on the edge of the bank and threw a chunk of wood into the lake. Jud got to it first and grabbed it. No sooner than he had the wood in his mouth, when a paw came down on his head pushing it under water. The wood floated up; Bugle grabbed it and brought it in.

Bugle liked to go ice fishing too and if there were any other fishermen around, he would sometimes have a fish before I finished cutting the first hole. I can still remember one fisherman on Shelburne Pond hollering, "He took my biggest one!" I could tell a lot of stories about Bugle, but I will just say that of all the dogs I have ever owned, he was the best.

Making a Break from New York City

Summer was coming to an end and the time had come to make the break from New York City. With my two years' experience as an electronic technician, I applied for three positions, all in Vermont and all within a 1½-hour drive to the camp. Conveniently, a bridge connected New York to Vermont just a few miles north of the camp.

Both IBM and General Electric offered me a job. I chose to work for General Electric at a firing range in Jericho. General Electric is noted for making light bulbs, refrigerators, and other appliances. Few people realize that back then GE also made guns—not your average hunting rifles—but mini-guns for the military. These six-barreled guns were driven by an electric motor and fired 100 rounds per second. Each one had to be tested. My job was to run the instrumentation to ascertain that voltages, currents, and starting and stopping times were within the specifications.

When I learned that mini-guns fired 7.62 mm bullets, the same caliber as a 308 hunting rifle, it didn't take me long to buy one. At that time, I was reloading ammo for several rifles and shotguns and thought I would make use of some of the empty brass at the firing range.

One day I saw a man at a bench pulling projectiles from bullets that had become damaged in a faulty system and dumping the powder into a box.

"What are you going to do with that powder? I asked.

"Burn it," he said.

"Not anymore," I said. "I will take all you have."

Working at the range had another bonus. A beautiful trout stream with large brown trout flowed through the valley where the range was located. They often tested guns on weekends, but not all weekends. I had some very good fishing on that stream.

While working for GE, I boarded at a house in Underhill, a short drive to work. Mrs. Parent was a good cook and she made breakfast and supper and fixed lunch for me and two other boarders. Her land had a stream on it where I could catch and keep live bait and woods to hunt in. Bugle had his house in the backyard.

Some say that the difference between a human and an animal is that an animal cannot reason. Well, I agree that an animal does not come close to reasoning like a human, but one day Bugle showed me that he reasoned enough to make a decision for himself. Bugle loved to hunt and the woods out in back was a temptation for him. One day, I was outside with him when I looked up and saw him quite a distance away heading for the woods at full speed. I hollered his name and he came to a full stop. He turned and looked at me and then looked at the woods. He made his decision and off to the woods he went!

Vermont offered some good fishing with streams and lakes within a short drive of the house. One time Mrs. Parent's son Robert, just out of the army, and I went ice fishing together. It was April and we had gotten some thaws and refreezes, the kind of weather that makes for good maple-syruping. It was a mile hike to the pond, and not realizing how much snow was still on the ground, I made a poor choice of footgear. I wore a pair of boots cut off from waders that had no shoelaces. The snow went over my boots and at every step the boot scooped up wet snow. My feet were freezing when we arrived at the pond, but that was not going to stop me from fishing on such a nice sunny day. I sat on a ledge, took off by boots and socks, wrung the water out of my socks, put them back on, and headed out onto the pond. The alternating thawing and freezing had created a foot of slush between a layer of crust on top and hard ice on the bottom. I tested the bottom layer of ice and found it to be safe. The crust was not strong enough to support my weight so I broke through it at every step. This was a bit disconcerting for my friend and he decided to stay on shore. Before I could cut the second hole, I caught the first trout and then several more in quick succession. It was some of the fastest trout fishing I have ever experienced, but even that did not entice Robert out onto the ice.

Chapter 5
An Important Decision

Your word is a lamp to my feet and a light to my path. - Psalm 119:105

Up until the age of 25, I had faithfully attended Sunday Mass. One sunny day, I was in church looking out the window. I thought: *Am I in church because I want to or because I have to?*

The truthful answer: *because I had to.*

I had been taught that missing mass was a mortal sin and if I should die before confessing a mortal sin to a priest, I would burn in hell forever. I realized that what kept me going to church was fear of burning forever. I thought that that was not a good motive, so that day I decided to stop going to church.

Although I had been taught a lot in my 13 years of Christian education, I did not really understand the gospel—the good news about salvation through Jesus *alone*. It was not until I started reading the Bible sometime later that I began understanding the gospel.

The Bible tells us that we all have sinned and deserve death (Romans 3:23; 6:23). But because of His great love for us and His great mercy, Jesus took the penalty of our sins and died in our place. "While we were still sinners, Christ died for us" (Romans 5:8). We are saved by God's grace (unmerited favour) through faith (by believing; Ephesians 2:8). Eternal life is *completely* God's gift to us (Ephesians 2:8); we cannot add anything to it. If we had something to add, we would be boasting about it and this would open us up to pride, the sin that led to Lucifer's downfall (Ezekiel 28:17) and eventually to all the suffering and death in this world.

We receive salvation the *moment* we believe and accept Jesus as our Lord and Saviour. Jesus said, "He who believes in Me *has* everlasting life" (John 6:47; emphasis mine). We are saved at that moment! Salvation is not based on anything we do; it is a legal transaction, an instantaneous accounting change in Heaven's Book of Life. The apostle Paul put it this way: "But to him who does not work but believes on Him who justifies the ungodly, his faith is *accounted* for righteousness" (Romans 4:5). Paul goes on to say, "Therefore, having been justified by faith, we have peace with God through our Lord Jesus Christ" (Romans 5:1). Read this paragraph again and let this incredible good news sink in.

When we really take this home, we will love God with all our heart and have a desire to please Him and carry out His plan for our lives. We will want everyone we meet to have eternal life too and will be looking for ways to share what we know and Who we know with others. We will gladly accept the great commission of taking the gospel to every kindred, tongue, and people (Matthew 28:19, 20). The things of this world that have attracted us will lose their attraction. As long as we keep looking to Jesus and asking Him for His Holy Spirit each day, we will gradually become more like Him. By beholding Him, we will be changed (2 Corinthians 3:18).

We should understand that sanctification (becoming more like Jesus) is the work of a lifetime and we will always be advancing. As the apostle Paul put it, we should always be "pressing toward that goal" (Philippians 3:14). The psalmist wrote: "Your word is a lamp to my feet and a light to my path" (Psalm 119:105). As the Holy Spirit lightens our path with new truths, we will continually be advancing. And we can be confident "that He who has begun a good work in you will complete it until the day of Jesus Christ" (Philippians 1:6).

As we are advancing on the lighted path of God's word, we will probably fall and sin. When that happens, the devil will try to keep us down. He will tell us we will never make it. *Do not believe him!* The devil is a liar and the father of lies (John 8:44). The true word of God says: "If we confess our sins, He is faithful and just to forgive us our sins and to cleanse us from all unrighteousness" (1 John 1:9). *Never give up!* As long as we are sincere in confessing a sin and repent (wanting to turn away from it), God's promise (1 John 1:9) to forgive us holds true. When Peter asked Jesus how many times he should forgive his brother who sinned against him and suggested up to seven times, Jesus answered, "I tell you not seven times, but seventy times seven" (Matthew 18:21, 22). God will do no less for us.

To become a "new creation," restored to the image of God, we need knowledge, understanding, and wisdom. Bible knowledge is superior to any other kind of knowledge. It tells us how to have eternal life. Speaking through the prophet Hosea, God said, "My people are destroyed from lack of knowledge" (Hosea 4:6).

Understanding takes knowledge a step farther. When God was leading the Israelites into the Promised Land, He spoke to His people through Moses about His commandments: "You shall bind them [God's commandments] as a sign on your hand, and they shall be as frontlets between your eyes" (Deuteronomy 6:8). Some people have taken this command literally and put the written commandments in a little box, called a phylactery, and wear it on their foreheads. They have knowledge of what God said, but do not understand what He meant. God meant for His commandments to be put in their minds. In order to understand the meaning behind the words, before reading, we must ask God for His Holy Spirit, the Spirit of Truth (John 14:17; 15:26). The apostle Paul wrote: "But the natural man does not receive the things of the Spirit of God, for they are foolishness to him; nor can he know them, because they are spiritually discerned" (1 Corinthians 2:14).

As important as knowledge and understanding are, without wisdom they are worthless! Jesus told a parable that explains what it means to be wise: "Therefore whoever hears these sayings of Mine, and *does them*, I will liken him to a *wise* man who built his house on the rock: and the rain descended, the floods came, and the winds blew and beat on that house; and it did not fall, for it was founded on the rock. But everyone who hears these sayings of Mine, and does not do them, will be like a foolish man who built his house on the sand: and the rain descended, the floods came, and the winds blew and beat on that house; and it fell. And great was its fall" (Matthew 7:24–27; emphasis mine).

In Old Testament times, God said the same thing to the prophet

Ezekiel: "So they come to you as people do, they sit before you as My people, and they hear your words, but they *do not do them*; for with their mouth they show much love, but their hearts pursue their own gain" (Ezekiel 33:31; emphasis mine). Wisdom is putting into practice what we know and understand.

As I am writing this, a verse is coming to my mind which God impressed me with when I first started reading the Bible. I read it at my baptism: "How much better to get wisdom than gold! And to get understanding is to be chosen rather than silver" (Proverbs 16:16). At that time I thought it was simply saying that Biblical *understanding* and *wisdom* were more valuable than precious metals worth a lot of money. Now I understand that it says even more. Understanding—knowing what God would have us do—is better than silver, but wisdom—actually doing it—is better than gold!

Chapter 6

Back to School

Wine is a mocker, strong drink is a brawler, and whoever is led astray by it is not wise. - Proverbs 20:1

General Electric sold the mini-guns to the government on contracts and it was either boom or bust. In 1970 a bust was coming, pink slips were being given out, and I knew mine was coming.

The University of Vermont was in Burlington, fifteen miles away and I heard they had a program in wildlife management, something I never knew existed when graduating from high school. One of the benefits of my military service was being able to go to school on the GI Bill. I visited the university, talked to a wildlife professor, and decided to start that coming fall. I attended school like it was a job, leaving in the morning and coming home at night. When I did not have classes, I was studying in the library. Some of my previous college courses shortened my time by one semester. I graduated in December 1973.

I knew that I was in a competitive field with employment being limited mostly to state and federal agencies so I made it a point to obtain experience in work-related summer jobs. In the first summer I worked at the Dead Creek Waterfowl Refuge in Addison, Vermont. The refuge was just across the bridge from the camp, so I was able to stay at the camp with my mother and commute from there.

My work consisted of plowing, harrowing, and planting crops for the geese. I also helped band geese and ducks. To catch ducks, we set traps in the impoundments and baited them with corn. We moved the four-by-eight-foot traps by balancing them across a square-ended canoe powered by a small outboard motor. We banded wood ducks by gliding up to a wood duck box, quickly sticking a paddle handle in the entrance hole, and then reaching through the top door to remove and band the mother duck. We banded Canada Geese by rounding them up in a goose drive when they were molting and not able to fly.

In my second summer, I worked for the New York Pollution Unit in East Avon, New York. We collected and identified macroinvertebrates (e.g., stoneflies, mayflies, and caddis flies) in streams to assess the water quality. Macroinvertebrates can be better indicators of water quality than water samples because macroinvertebrates live in the stream for extended periods as opposed to a water sample which could miss a brief toxic discharge. We also conducted on-site bioassays in streams using minnows in cages. The macroinvertebrate monitoring led to the discovery of a water treatment plant discharging chlorine into a stream and the minnow bioassay led to a construction site that was allowing a petroleum product to enter a nearby stream.

The School of Hard Knocks

Soon after my arrival in East Avon, I decided to go to a movie. The air-conditioned theater would provide some relief from the summer heat. Before going in, I drank one or two bottles of beer. When I came out of the cool movie theater into the warm air, I felt a little woozy. It was now dark, and I headed home. On the way home, I saw a yellow light ahead and came to a stop. Almost immediately I was hit in the rear. It was not a hard hit, and no one was hurt with both cars receiving only minor damage. It turned out that the yellow light was not a signal light, but an overhead mercury light that had a yellow color. A policeman showed up and wrote a report. I explained the reason why I stopped and that I was new to the area. He never questioned that I was under the influence and did not give me a ticket, but I knew that the alcohol I had consumed prior to the movie had clouded my judgment and had contributed to the accident. That was the only time that I have stopped for an overhead street light, but I have to say it was not the only time that my mind has been impaired by alcohol.

For about thirty years I have been going to the Jefferson County Jail to study the Bible with the inmates. I would estimate that over 95 percent of the people I study with are in jail for reasons directly or indirectly related to alcohol and/or drugs. Driving under the Influence (DUI), hitting pedestrians and bicyclists, resisting arrest, assault, and stealing are often associated with alcohol. But the worst alcohol-related tragedy I am aware of involved two brothers, both friends of mine. Drinking beer was a large part of both their lives. Now one is dead from a bullet to the head and the other is in prison. So much heartache could be avoided if people would heed the words of the wise man Solomon, "Wine is a mocker, strong drink is a brawler, and whoever is led astray by it is not wise" (Proverbs 20:1).

There is a saying, "Everything in moderation." But this is not true. For substances like alcohol, abstinence is the best way to go. Some will say people in the Bible drank wine. Even Jesus changed water into wine at the wedding in Cana (John 2:1–10). Yes, He did, but it was unfermented sweet grape juice. When Jesus hung on the cross suffering excruciating pain and was offered wine mixed with gall, He refused to drink it (Matthew 27:34).

It is important that we keep our minds in good working condition so that we will always think clearly. In the last days, which I believe we are in, people will receive on/in their foreheads either the "seal of God" (Revelation 7:3; 9:4; 13:16) or the dreaded "mark of the beast" (Revelation 14:9; 20:4). This seal or mark is not some kind of tattoo or implanted chip. It refers to our thinking, our choices, who we are, and who we give our allegiance to. Ultimately, there are only two choices: God or Satan.

The Bible uses the same word "wine" for both fermented and unfermented grape juice. We need to consider the context in order to tell which one it is. Some may say medical research has shown that wine is good for the heart. The phytochemicals in wine are good for the heart, but we can benefit from the same phytochemicals in unfermented, sweet grape juice without the harmful effects of the alcohol. "Therefore, whether you eat or drink, or whatever you do, do all to the glory of God" (1 Corinthians 10:31). If you are interested in learning more on the subject of wine in the Bible, read Samuele Bacchiocci's book, *Wine in the Bible.*[1]

More Summer Adventures

During my third summer and also after I graduated in December 1973, I worked at the Special Studies Unit of the New York Conservation Department in Ray Brook, New York. The Conservation Department was stocking Lake Champlain with landlocked Atlantic salmon, lake trout, and steelhead, and wanted to assess the population of lamprey in the lake.

Lamprey are parasitic fish that attach themselves to the side of a fish, gnaw through the skin with their rasping teeth, and suck the fish's blood, sometimes killing their host. Similar to trout and salmon, lamprey migrate up tributary streams at spawning time. Larval lamprey, called ammocetes, spend seven to nine years in the soft stream bottom before going into the lake and attaching to fish.

I was part of an electrofishing crew shocking lamprey in Lake Champlain tributaries to determine their abundance. One time, while trout fishing Putts Creek, I observed a spawning pair building a nest in a riffle. Unlike a salmon or trout which uses its tail to dig a redd (nest), a lamprey constructs a nest by picking up and moving stones with its mouth.

I also helped trap and spawn wild brook trout and I conducted a winter creel census on Lake Champlain using a snowmobile. One time the ice had a layer of water on it, making it very slippery. When checking some fishermen, I walked and slid a distance from the machine to reach them. When I tried to walk back to the snowmobile against the wind, the wind blew me farther away and I ended up having to crawl back to the snowmobile. Conducting the creel census and lamprey survey had fringe benefits; I learned some good fishing places!

Pursuing a Childhood Dream

Before I started work that last summer of 1973, I was able to fulfill (as it turned out, almost fulfill) a dream I had in childhood. Growing up, my two favourite magazines were *Outdoor Life* and *Field and Stream*. In one of those magazines I read about a fishing trip on the Hudson

River that always stayed in my mind.

You may picture the Hudson River as a large river separating New York from New Jersey and having ocean-going ships. However, like all rivers the Hudson River starts small. Its origin is 250 miles north in the Adirondack Mountains. The article I read was about a twenty-eight-mile fishing trip through a wilderness area from Newcomb to North Creek. The brown trout caught on this trip were described as having red spots the size of dimes. That was enough for me to remember it years later!

When school ended in May, I persuaded another student to go with me. The only boat I had was a Sears and Roebuck twelve-foot fiberglass Gamefisher. Besides fishing gear, we brought along sleeping bags and other camping supplies and a topographic map. For lifejackets, we had seat cushions with arm loops.

Where we launched in Newcomb the river was flat with no rapids. My topographic map showed Ord Falls ahead and I was keeping an eye out for it. We used the oars in the normal fashion in the flat water stretch, but when the river started dropping, we used them like paddles with Mike in the bow and me in the stern. After a while I realized we must have passed through Ord Falls. It was not a vertical drop like some waterfalls, but only steep rapids.

I cannot remember exactly how many times the boat overturned, but early on in the trip, I spotted something orange on the shore which turned out to be a life jacket. It was an old, cork-filled kind, but at this point it was looking pretty good to me. Mike and I discussed who should wear it and since he was a card-carrying lifeguard and I a marginal swimmer, we decided I should wear it.

The Gamefisher was getting pretty banged up on the rocks, so at our campsite we patched it with duct tape. In one particularly bad crack along the keel, I wedged in a sock. Our sleeping bags were double wrapped in garbage bags and were staying dry. However, we could never tie them in securely enough to stay in the boat when it overturned. Amazingly, we always found them farther downstream floating in an eddy.

Eventually, the damage to the boat was beyond patching. We were considering walking out when I spotted an aluminum rowboat upside down on the opposite shore. We decided the Gamefisher had enough left in her to make it across the river. We found the aluminum boat to be damaged, but not as badly as the Gamefisher. We transferred all our gear into the aluminum boat and made it farther down the river before the rapids and rocks damaged it beyond repair.

On the final dump, Mike and I swam to opposite sides of the river with the boat ending up on Mike's side, which was also the side closest to the nearest road. When I attempted to swim across to Mike's side, the current took me downstream a lot faster than I was going across. I ended up a little way from shore out of the current behind a huge boulder with vertical sides. I was a lot closer to the shore I started from than I was to the opposite shore, so I swam back to the shore I started from. There was still some snow in the woods and the water was very cold. I crawled up on the shore and lay there for a while catching my breath.

I did not want to get into that cold water again, but I knew I had to. I walked downstream where there was a longer stretch between rapids. Mike did the same on his side, but since his side had a vertical cliff coming down to the water's edge, he had to climb up, bypass the cliff and come back down. Mike found a long stick and positioned himself just upstream from the rapids I would be heading toward. I got as far upstream as I could below the upstream rapids and started swimming for all I was worth as the current swept me rapidly downstream. Just as I was about to enter the rapids, I grabbed the end of Mike's stick and he pulled me ashore.

We changed into the driest clothes we had, made a stretcher using the oars to carry our gear and started walking toward the road several miles away. We ran onto a trail that led us to some cabins. By that time, it was getting dark and a cold rain was falling. Being cold and wet, we decided to break into one of the cabins. Once inside, we looked for blankets. Mike found one in a container, but his hands were too cold to work the zipper. Just then we heard a vehicle and went outside. It was the caretaker of the church camp we were at. We apologized for breaking into the cabin and he was very nice about it and said it happens all the time by boaters needing to walk out. He said they called that stretch of river the "graveyard." We had been seeing parts of boats along the riverbanks. Using his phone, I called my mother at the camp and she came and rescued us. We never did do any fishing on this trip.

In retrospect, taking a rowboat down that river, besides not having lifejackets, was crazy. In canoeing terms, the river was Class 3[+]. I have always felt that finding that life jacket just where and when I needed it was providential—another instance of God's protective hand over me.

Time for Change

Part way through the school year, my mother was coming home after a day of work at the blood bank. As she was about to enter her door on the third floor landing of the apartment building, a mugger grabbed her purse. My mother fell, but she did not stay down. She got up, chased the mugger down the stairs, down the block, and around the corner. The chase ended when he ran into a basketball court and climbed over a chain link fence.

After that incident I decided it was time for my mother to leave New York City. I found a house in Shelburne, Vermont and moved my mother there where we lived together until I finished school. It was a good location for both of us. It was near the university and it was only a one-hour drive to the camp. When I graduated, my mother found a house in Crown Point, which was only a ten-minute drive to the camp.

While attending school I saw something on the bulletin board that interested me. It was an advertisement to go to the University of Fairbanks on a research assistantship working on humpback whitefish. It was not the humpback whitefish that interested me so much as simply going to Alaska for some real fishing. Somehow after seeing that advertisement, I was certain I would be going. However, I was not accepted, but it did put an idea in my mind about going to graduate school.

1. Bacchiocchi, S. 1989. *Wine in the Bible: A Biblical Study on the Use of Alcoholic Beverages*, Biblical Perspectives, Berrien Springs, Michigan. Read it on line at:
http://www.anym.org/pdf/wine_in_the_Bible_samuele_bacchiocchi.pdf

Chapter 7
University of Maine

Deliver my soul, O Lord, from lying lips and from a deceitful tongue. -
Psalm 120:2

The Special Studies Unit in Ray Brook was looking for a boat for Lake Champlain's cold-water fishery program. When I heard they were planning to go to Maine to look for a boat, I asked to go along and visit the University of Maine at Orono where there was a Cooperative Fishery Unit. I met with the leader of the unit and discovered that they had a research assistantship for a project that I was a good match for. The research project was to determine if alewives competed with smelt for food in Echo Lake in Acadia National Park. This would involve identifying and comparing the stomach contents of hundreds of smelt and alewives. At the University of Vermont, I had completed a three-semester honors project in which I identified the stomach contents of several species of fish from Lake Champlain.

I applied, was accepted, and started school in 1974. I used bottom and mid-water trawls and a gill net set under the ice to capture the smelt and alewives. Smelt are negatively phototropic which means they are repelled by light. They feed on the bottom during the day and come up into the water column at night to feed on zooplankton, which are also negatively phototropic. Alewives are pelagic, meaning they remain in the water column all the time. Both feed on zooplankton and I became pretty good at identifying copepods and cladocerans by the time I finished looking at the stomach contents of about 1,500 fish. When I was not catching smelt and alewives in Echo Lake, I angled for the landlocked Atlantic salmon and rainbow trout there. Besides Echo Lake, I enjoyed fishing many other lakes and rivers during my two years in Maine. And I enjoyed hunting deer, snowshoe rabbits, grouse, woodcock, and ducks.

To better take advantage of the lakes and rivers surrounding me, I decided to get a boat, and Old Town, home of the famous Old Town canoes, was the next town over from Orono. I went to the factory.

I asked the salesman, "What is the toughest canoe you have?"

"Royalex, a composite material of ABS foam sandwiched between two layers of vinyl." The salesman took a 10-inch square piece of Royalex, leaned it up against something, and gave it a hard blow with a hammer. It flew across the room, and upon retrieving it, we found a dent on one side, but the other side unscathed. That convinced me and that day I bought a 17-foot Tripper model.

A friend and I took it out on the Stillwater River, a branch of the Penobscot River, for its maiden voyage. As its name implies the Stillwater is flat water with no rapids, but that did not stop us from dumping! We managed to get hung up on a rock just below the surface and over we went.

I did a lot of fishing and duck hunting from that boat on rivers and lakes during my two years in Maine and it still serves us well in Washington 40 years later.

Lying to the Judge

The law in Maine required that a hunter dress in fluorescent orange. I had always worn red to be visible to other hunters and thought that was sufficient. While walking down a woods road, gun in hand, I was stopped and ticketed by a game warden for not wearing orange. I had to appear in court. Before appearing, I thought of a way to avoid paying a fine. When the warden stopped me, I was walking on the road, not actually hunting. I would tell the judge I was not hunting, but on my way hunting. This was not entirely true because I had already been hunting before coming out to the road. In my heart, I knew it was a lie; my conscience was letting me know that. But I told a lie to avoid paying the fine.

is something that still comes up in my memory today and I am sorry I did it. I wish I would have told the truth and paid the fine.

The wise man Solomon said, "Lying lips are an abomination to the Lord, but those who deal truthfully are His delight" (Proverbs 12:22). God hates lying and any kind of deception. The eighth commandment tells us not to bear false witness (Exodus 20:16). Eve's believing Satan's lie, "You will not surely die," is what brought death and suffering to planet earth. Before that, Satan's lies deceived one third of all the angels in Heaven and caused them to be cast to the earth with him. Revelation 12:9 says: "So the great dragon was cast out, that serpent of old, called the Devil and Satan, who deceives the whole world; he was cast to the earth, and his angels were cast out with him." Revelation 12:4 tells us that he cast them out with his tail: "His tail drew a third of the stars (angels, Rev 1:20) of heaven and threw them to the earth." Isaiah 9:15 says: "The prophet who teaches lies, he is the tail." Satan lied about God's loving, other-centered character, and painted God with his own unloving, self-centered character. One-third of all the angels bought his "tall tail."

Unfortunately, a lot of us humans have also bought into Satan's lies about God's character. A major part of Jesus' taking on human flesh and living among us was to reveal who God, our Father, really is or more aptly put "what He is like." To know what God is like, we only have to look at the life of Jesus as recorded in the writings of Matthew, Mark, Luke, and John. When Philip asked Jesus to show him the Father, Jesus said to him, "Have I been with you so long, and yet you have not known Me, Philip? He who has seen Me has seen the Father; so how can you say, 'Show us the Father?'" (John 14:9). Jesus is the "brightness of His [the Father's] glory, and the express image of His person" (Hebrews 1:3).

Not all people have bought into Satan's deception about the character of God. The disciple John wrote about God's children who will know Him: "Beloved, now we are children of God; and it has not yet been revealed what we shall be, but we know that when He is revealed, we shall be like Him, for we shall see Him as He is" (1 John 3:2). Revelation calls this group of people the "144,000." They have God's name (character) "written on their foreheads" (Revelation 14:1) and "no deceit" comes out of their mouths (Revelation 14:5). Ultimately, there will be no liars in God's kingdom (Revelation 21:27; 22:15).

Chapter 8
Moving to Washington

Jesus answered and said to her, "Whoever drinks of this water will thirst again, but whoever drinks of the water that I shall give him will never thirst. But the water that I shall give him will become in him a fountain of water springing up into everlasting life" - John 4:13, 14

As my graduation from the University of Maine neared, I applied for work. I applied to the U.S. Fish and Wildlife Service for every position I was qualified for. I started hearing about jobs all over the country, but none interested me until I heard about one in Washington State. What interested me more than the work was its rural location on the Olympic Peninsula. With my course work, fieldwork, and laboratory work completed and only my thesis to write, I applied for and obtained the position of fishery biologist. In December 1976, I loaded up my Toyota Corolla station wagon with all my fishing poles, guns, and canoe and headed west. Ten days later I arrived in Washington.

I was fortunate to find a place to live on Kilisut Harbor just a few miles south of Marrowstone Field Station where I would be working. The owners of the house were taking a year to drive around the country and were looking for a house sitter. I was not there long when I bought Jake, a black lab puppy. Jake loved the water and loved to retrieve including any shoes he could find from the next-door neighbors. I trained him to retrieve on hand signals and Jake and I had a lot of fun hunting ducks together. Before the owners returned, I bought a ten-by-fifty-foot mobile home and set it up on property just down the shoreline from where I was living.

Marrowstone Field Station is located on the northern tip of Marrowstone Island located off the northeast corner of the Olympic Peninsula where the Strait of Juan de Fuca joins Puget Sound. The field station was originally a light keeper's house. When things became automated, the Coast Guard gave the property to the Fish and Wildlife Service. It was a wonderful place to work. Looking out the window, I often saw seals, killer whales, eagles, osprey, and blacktail deer. I caught salmon by casting off the beach right outside the door.

The field station existed mainly for the purpose of conducting bioassays on salmon in their smoltification stage when they transition from fresh water to salt water. Most fish would die attempting this, but salmon were designed with the ability to maintain an optimum blood salt level whether in fresh or salt water, a process known as osmoregulation.

Fish, like other animals raised in crowded conditions, are susceptible to disease. It is sometimes necessary to treat hatchery fish with antibiotics before releasing them. Although the treated fish may appear healthy upon release, it is unknown if the antibiotics affect the salmon's ability to osmoregulate.

The wet lab at the field station, plumbed with both fresh and salt water, was designed to simulate the change from fresh to salt water. Experiments were conducted in which salmon were treated with different antibiotics, brought through smoltification, and observed for a period of time afterward.

I was not part of this research. I worked in a branch of the Service called Fisheries Assistance. Project leader, Cliff Bosley, and I assisted other branches of the Service, Indian tribes, and other organizations in matters relating to water quality.

My first duty was to set up a water quality lab under Cliff's guidance. Cliff had retired from Wyoming Game and Fish and had done similar work there. We set the lab up in what was once the living room of the light keeper's house. Benches along three walls provided space for the laboratory equipment. A chimney on the fourth wall was ideal for venting our flame atomic absorption spectrophotometer used for heavy metal analysis. We stored chemical reagents in the one-time pantry and set up an analytical balance there. The balance could only be used on calm days because wind against the side of the building made it unstable.

During my first few years at the field station, Cliff and I assisted Indian tribes. On one occasion, we assisted the Warm Springs Indian Tribe in Oregon where an infestation of spruce budworm had broken out. Spruce budworm, the larval stage of a moth, was severely damaging the coniferous trees on the reservation. To suppress the infestation, a plan was made to spray the trees with Sevin-4-oil, a carbaryl insecticide. Because Sevin-4-oil is toxic to aquatic organisms, the stream in the spray area was to be protected by a no-spray buffer on both sides. We were to assess the spraying by monitoring macroinvertebrates and fish in the stream.

We collected macroinvertebrate samples from riffles before, immediately after, and several months after the spraying. We also set up drift nets that captured macroinvertebrates drifting in the current before and during the spraying. And we collected rainbow trout after the spraying and had them analyzed for acetylcholinesterase. Sevin-4-oil is known to affect the nervous system by inhibiting acetylcholinesterase.

Based on the large number of macroinvertebrates in the drift samples during spraying and a reduction in the number of macroinvertebrates in the riffles after the spraying, we concluded that the insecticide had drifted into the stream and was detrimental to the macroinvertebrate population. No impairment was discerned in the trout; their acetylcholinesterase levels tested normal.

During our stay on the reservation, I helped the tribal fishery biologist plant trout by airplane into some high mountain lakes. Surrounded by juvenile trout in water-filled plastic bags, I knelt in the rear of the aircraft next to a small window. The pilot would swoop low over a lake, and on his signal, I would empty the bag out the window. Before we finished, the rubber band came off one of the bags and I had a lot of fish flopping around me. I managed to brush a fair number of them out the window on a pass over the lake. However, I did find a few in one of my boots after we landed.

After a few years, my main work shifted to visiting federal fish hatcheries in the Northwest and analyzing their water sources, which could be a stream, well, or combination of both. When fish began dying at the Eagle Creek National Fish Hatchery in Oregon, I analyzed their water and found it to contain high levels of cadmium. It turned out that they had recently installed new valves in their recirculating fish tanks. The valves turned out to be cadmium-plated. Cadmium is extremely toxic to fish even at very low concentrations.

Other work included collecting fish in the Columbia, Snake, and Rogue rivers for contaminant analysis under the National Pesticides Monitoring Program, controling carp on waterfowl refuges, and assisting the Washington fishery biologist by analyzing water from local streams. My job included field work, lab work, and report writing, and I enjoyed the variety.

Chapter 9
Married at Last

And the Lord God said, "It is not good that man should be alone." -
Genesis 2:18

Unlike today when canoes and kayaks are commonly seen on car tops, I do not remember seeing any during my first six months on the Olympic Peninsula. Someone mentioned that I should check the bulletin board at the REI store in Seattle. I did just that and discovered the Paddle Trails Canoe Club. I called the number listed and the person answering the call referred me to Linda Petrie.

Before continuing, I will divulge something about myself. I am an extremely shy, introverted person. That's the way I started life. From my teen years and even before, I was attracted to girls, but it pretty much just stayed an attraction. For one thing, about the only thing I knew how to talk about was fish! In high school, I never went to dances and never went on a date. My college years were not much better. Once I took a girl bullhead fishing where I used to work on the Dead Creek Waterfowl Refuge, but the fish were not biting, and she wasn't either.

Now at 33 years of age in Washington, I was still hoping things would change. I called Linda's number and she answered the phone. That in itself was unusual because Linda was an avid canoeist and it was very unusual for her to be home to answer the phone. Normally she would have been out canoeing. Linda built her first canoe and went canoeing every weekend and even went after work. But providentially she was home when I called, and we made plans to canoe the Skykomish River. That was the first of many times paddling together.

Linda didn't mind if I talked about fish. I think she liked hearing my fishing stories. And she says that I really impressed her with my fishing ability when we paddled the Sol Duc River. I was in the bow with my fishing pole in hand while Linda skilfully guided the canoe down the river.

I would casually say, "Bound to be a trout under that log over there," and would cast over and catch one.

I really liked Linda whose name means "beautiful" and it fit Linda perfectly. Linda is as beautiful on the inside as she is on the outside. A year after our first paddle together, on June 3, 1978, we were married on my front lawn. In beautiful calligraphy Linda wrote the invitation on green paper. Besides the where and when, it read, "Picnic Buffet follows the wedding. Canoeing, volleyball, and baseball games continue all day. Dress comfortably and casually. Please bring a chair, cushion, or blanket for relaxing, enjoying friends and fresh air." One of our wedding guests framed the invitation in an artistic wooden frame and gave it to us as a wedding present.

We played softball at the wedding and just had a good time. My mother made an eight-foot-long wedding cake; she made it in sections and glued it together with frosting. We cut the first piece with a canoe paddle. We had clam chowder in a large navy pot, heated with briquettes. We also had smoked sturgeon, which Cliff and I had caught on the Columbia River for pesticide analysis. We only needed a little bit for the analysis and we could not see the rest of it going to waste.

Linda was well known in the canoe club and a lot of her paddling friends came to the wedding. They joined together to give us a grain grinder, which we still use regularly forty years later. Every Sunday morning Linda asks me, "Do you want anything special for breakfast?"

I reply, "How about some pancakes?"

And Linda grinds up some whole-wheat flour and makes pancakes.

On our honeymoon we camped on the Elwha River. We found an island made by a small side channel branching off the main stem. We reached the island by walking on a fallen log across the side channel. It was a beautiful camping spot with grass and moss and a scattering of big leaf maples. We watched a mother harlequin duck trying to coax her newly hatched ducklings from the quiet side channel into the fast moving main stem. She must have succeeded because a while later they were gone. I caught some trout and an interesting thing happened when I was cleaning them on the riverbank. Through the river's cloudy glacial till, I could see something shiny on the river bottom. Curious, I reached in and pulled it out. It was Linda's wedding ring! She was unaware of losing it.

Paddling Style

Linda may have been impressed with my fishing style, but she sure wasn't impressed with my paddling style. On the Sol Duc River trip my paddle got wedged in some rocks and I lost my grip on it. Linda claims that it just flew out of my hands as my paddle was looking more like a whirling helicopter blade as I constantly switched sides.

Now I need to explain. I have been in boats all my life and when I bought the Old Town Tripper, I just went out and started using it. I used it on lots of Maine rivers. I never went to canoeing school like Linda had. To me switching from one side to the other was perfectly natural. Linda did not see it that way. She had been taught to stay on one side and only switch when you became tired. Eventually, we worked things out.

Working things out came after canoeing the Yakima River in eastern Washington. We were swiftly shooting down the river with me in the bow and Linda in the stern when all of a sudden Linda was going down the river on her own, along side the boat! I do not know how she exited the canoe without me noticing. When we made it to shore and I asked her what happened, she said she could not stand my switching anymore and was either going to hit me on the head with the paddle or jump out. I am glad she jumped out! I still did not see anything wrong with my switching style and came up with a plan to work things out. I would try it her way for one year and she would try it my way for a year, and then we would decide. After a year of paddling without switching, I became used to it and we never did try it my way. Recently, I learned a saying that I already knew intuitively, "Happy wife, happy life."

A Woman of Many Talents

Linda is a person of many talents. Her cooking ability is well known in our community. She knits, crochets, and weaves with ease, but her real expertise is in growing things. Linda's knowledge of seeds and growing them into flowers and vegetables exceeds my knowledge about fish and catching them. Most recently she was showing me tiny seeds that she collected from her carnivorous pitcher plants and venous fly traps.

Unlike my personality, Linda has a warmth about her that attracts people. She cannot go grocery shopping without meeting people she knows. Kids especially like her. Linda grew up in 4-H and has been a 4-H leader since I have known her. The kids come to our house now for gardening, cooking, and sewing. Often the kids come away learning more than the basic subject. As she sees a need, she fills it. It might be in math, history, or geography.

Besides our garden in the backyard, Linda has a garden at the Cedarbrook Early Learning Center where she teaches gardening to the little children. I am sure she has instilled a love for gardening into many little minds. As an occupational therapist working with special-needs children for many years, Linda has a way with children and would have made an excellent schoolteacher.

You may have heard it said that God always answers our prayers. Sometimes He says "yes"; sometimes He says "no"; and sometimes he says "wait." When, as a young man, I prayed for a wife, God said "wait." I can honestly say that Linda was worth the wait. I could not have found a better wife if I scoured the entire planet.

Soon we were blessed with a baby girl who we named Dawn. We started early to introduce Dawn to canoeing, camping, and fishing. Dawn must have inherited mostly her mother's genes. She is sociable in the extreme and is well liked in this small community. She also inherited Linda's artistic talents. Dawn could sit across the table from you and sketch your face in five minutes. She also takes some amazing pictures with her cell phone/camera. Dawn found her niche as a hairstylist which turned out to be a good deal for me and Linda and I get my hair cut right in my kitchen. After sampling city life in Seattle and Portland,

Dawn decided a small community is the best place to live and settled in Port Townsend.

Heather joined the family three and one-half years after Dawn. Heather is the serious, studious type. She went to many different schools, and following in her mother's footsteps, ended up with a PhD in occupational therapy. Heather could have been a financial manager. No one can sniff out a better deal than Heather. Heather learned how to fly while in high school before she got her driver's license. She has done some hang gliding and, of course, knows how to handle a paddle. She married Nigel Standish and they live with their two boys Conrad and Griffin in Nigel's home state of Virginia.

When Nigel met Heather, he was in the Air Force teaching survival school. More specifically, he was a SERE trainer. SERE stands for Survival, Evasion, Resistance, and Escape. His trainees were given a live rabbit and a chicken to survive on for a week in the woods of northeast Washington. Any other food was obtained using survival skills. Recently, Nigel told me how he caught trout in a stream on a double-pointed-ended stick. I am still not exactly sure how he did it.

His best story puts my story of "catching" a grouse to shame. When Nigel was being trained as a SERE, a grouse flew low over his head and he quickly reached up and caught it! When his four years were up, he went to the University of Virginia and obtained a PhD in Education. He is now the Director of STEM for the schools in Charlottesville. STEM, which stands for Science, Technology, Engineering, and Mathematics, is an integrated approach to learning.

Chapter 10
Discouraged

For consider Him who endured such hostility from sinners against Himself, lest you become weary and discouraged in your souls. - Hebrews 12:3

When I stopped going to church, I never stopped believing in God, but I cannot say that I had a real relationship with God. I do not recall praying that much, but two things came together to change that. One was the thought that came to me once in a while: *how will I raise my children concerning religion?*

The second was the discouragement I was feeling due to an increasing awareness of how badly our environment is contaminated, and in particular, fish. At the University of Vermont I had written a paper on the effects of the insecticide DDT on wildlife and at the University of Maine I had written one on the effects of organophosphate pesticides on fish. I had no idea I would be learning about contaminants first hand.

In writing a report on the sturgeon that we sampled in the Columbia River, I was mainly interested in the contaminants' effect on the sturgeon population. Based on a literature review of the effects of contaminants on other species of fish, I concluded that the polychlorinated biphenyls (PCBs) and other contaminants found in the sturgeon could impair the sturgeon's reproductive ability. However, the literature review revealed more than that. I started seeing studies that related contaminants in fish to cancer and birth defects in humans. It was an eye opener!

Of all the food groups, fish are the most susceptible to accumulating contaminants because of the long food chain in the aquatic environment. Each time a fish eats a smaller fish, its burden of contaminants is passed on to the larger fish, a process known as bioaccumulation. Actually, the process starts even earlier in the food chain with zooplankton, the food of small fish. It is usually the larger fish that people eat such as tuna, sword fish, and bass that have the highest concentrations.

State health agencies and the U.S. Environmental Protection Agency post fish advisories warning people, especially children and women of child-bearing age, about contaminants in fish. The advisories warn consumers: not to eat certain kinds of fish anywhere; not to eat any kind of fish from certain water bodies; and to limit their consumption of all kinds of fish wherever they are caught. Find out what the advisories say in your state by Googling "fish advisories" and the name of your state.

All of this was weighing on my mind. I consider myself an optimist, but I am also a realist. In many ways I could see the world, environmentally speaking, going downhill and I did not think that we humans were able to fix it. Like the side effects that accompany medications, a lot of what we do for good purposes have *unintended consequences*.

We build dams to generate hydroelectric power and block migrating salmon. We build nuclear power plants and they blow up (Chernobyl, Ukraine) and spread radiation on the land or they are destroyed by a tsunami (Fukushima, Japan) and contaminate the water. We build nuclear storage sites (Hanford, Washington) and the containers leak. We burn coal and cause acid rain and mercury fallout. We build offshore oil wells and they pollute the water. We develop fracking to extract more oil and cause earthquakes. We build oil pipelines to transport oil and the pipes leak and pollute soil and groundwater. We develop pesticides to increase crop yield and some cause birth defects and cancer. We develop chemicals (PCBs) to cool transformers and they too cause cancer and birth defects. Our track record speaks for itself.

Chapter 11

A New Discovery of an Old Book

Your word is a lamp to my feet and a light to my path. - Psalm 119:105

The question on my mind was: *Where is this world heading?* One day the thought came to me: "*The answer is in the Bible. Read the Bible.*" I mentioned my feelings about reading the Bible to Linda and one day she showed me an advertisement in the newspaper about a seminar on the book of Daniel. I did not know anything about the book of Daniel other than that it was in the Bible. I started going to the seminar and when it was over ten weeks later, Pastor Skip McClannahan asked me, "Do you want to study more?"

"Yes," I replied.

The pastor started coming to my house to study the Bible with me .

On one occasion he asked, "Do you want to accept Jesus as your Savior?"

I said, "Yes."

We knelt down and I asked Jesus to be my Savior.

During this time, I started reading the Bible, beginning at Genesis 1:1: "In the beginning, God created the heavens and the earth."

At about this time I was asked to assist the Spring Creek National Fish Hatchery on the Columbia River where they were having a problem called "soft shell." The salmon embryo was prematurely breaking through the shell membrane resulting in high mortality. While doing some experiments on the water that the eggs were hardened in, I stayed in an upstairs apartment in nearby Little White Salmon National Fish Hatchery. Reading the Bible was now a top priority and I purposely did not bring a TV or radio. Prior to going to the Daniel Seminar, I had started reading Louis L'Amour western books and I had just purchased two shopping bags full of his books. I was afraid they would distract me from reading the Bible, so I packaged them up and mailed them to my cousin Bill, who also liked Louis L'Amour.

Each day after work I would read the Bible. I was becoming more and more convinced that it was all true. However, there was one thing that bothered me and that was the length of time that life existed on earth. Based on the Bible's genealogy from Jesus to Adam, I estimated that Adam and all other life were created between 5,000 and 6,000 years ago. In six years of college I had been taught that life had been around for billions of years and that it started on its own from a simple cell that over time evolved into more complex life forms including us humans. Although I never gave evolution any credence, I was very much concerned about the long geologic time periods used to date fossils. My first thought was that the Bible's shorter time chronology was in error because it disagreed with the hard data obtained from radioactive dating. I spent a lot of time on my knees asking God for an answer to the time discrepancy.

Breakthrough

The first breakthrough came when I visited the Seventh-day Adventist Church in White Salmon, not far from where I was staying at the hatchery. While waiting for the service to start, I perused some books in the foyer. One jumped out at me: *Fossils, Flood, and Fire* by Harold Clark.[1] That was the beginning of God answering my prayers about the time discrepancy. I had read through the chapters in Genesis about the flood, but had not realized their importance. The next book I read that further opened my eyes was *The Genesis Flood* by John Whitcomb and Henry Morris.[2]

In a geology class I was taught uniformitarianism, the theory that changes in the earth's crust during geological history have resulted from the action of continuous and uniform processes. Based on this theory, the present is the key to the past.

For instance, by knowing the rate that the Colorado River is currently eroding the Grand Canyon and knowing how deep the Grand Canyon is, we can calculate the time it has taken the Grand Canyon to be carved out. Using rounded figures, if the erosion rate is 0.001 foot per year and the canyon is 6,000 feet deep, it would take 6,000,000 years to erode the canyon to its present depth. The problem with uniformitarianism is that it is based on the assumption that erosion has continued at a constant rate for 6,000,000 years. After much study, I believe that that assumption is false.

On a much smaller time scale, but representing the same principle, I have observed that it is not your average daily rainfall that alters the landscape. Rather it is an infrequent catastrophic event, such as a 100-year flood, that overnight changes the topography of the land. Marine fossils on mountain tops are evidence that water once covered those mountains. However, it is likely that the mountains were not as high at the time water covered them as they are today, and that uplifting has occurred. After examining the data through scientific eyes, I believe a catastrophic event, such as the worldwide flood described in Genesis 7 and 8, is a much better explanation of the geologic evidence than uniform change over a long period of time. It is not surprising that flood stories have been found among people cultures all over the world: Romans, Babylonians, Gypsies, Mongols, Africans, Australian Aborigines, Hindus, Polynesians, and American Indians. Dr. Richard André found and recorded eighty-eight flood stories.[3]

Assumptions

When animals die today, they soon disappear by consumption and decay. In order for animals to be preserved as fossils, they need to be buried rapidly in sediment as would occur in a catastrophic flood. Also, the sedimentary layers, such as those in the Grand Canyon, are flat as pancakes, one on top of the other and do not show signs of erosion. If each layer was exposed to weathering for long periods before the next layer was laid down, we would expect to see an uneven eroded surface.

Just as uniformitarianism is based on assumptions, radioactive dating and carbon dating methods are also based on assumptions. One assumption is that the decay rate is constant. Another is that none of the parent and daughter material (e.g., parent uranium to daughter lead) is missing.

True science is based on experimentation that can be replicated. We cannot do this with the million-year geologic time periods and verify the assumptions made in the radioactive dating method. I have noticed that assumptions tend to be overlooked.

Here is an example in my own field of fisheries. A fishery biologist needs to estimate the population of trout in a lake and uses the mark and recapture method. He sets nets and captures a number of trout. He counts and marks them with a tag or clipped fin and then releases them back into the lake. After a number of days, he sets his nets again and captures a number of trout, some of which will be marked and some of which will not be marked and he counts the number in each group. Using a formula based on proportions, he calculates the total population of trout in the lake and puts the estimate in his report. His estimate will be accurate *if* the following assumptions are met: 1) a sufficient amount of time elapsed between the two captures so that the marked fish were well mixed with the unmarked fish; 2) that the mortality rate for the marked and unmarked fish was the same during the time period between the two captures; and 3) that no fish entered or exited the lake from an inlet or outlet. If these assumptions are even mentioned, they take a back seat to the objective of the study—to obtain a population estimate. In reality, he has no way of knowing with certainty that all the assumptions were met.

I believe there are reasons why most, but not all, scientists believe that life on planet earth has existed for billions of years instead of thousands of years. If for whatever reason, one takes the view that there is no Creator God, the only other alternative is that life started by itself from atoms coming together to form something alive. And somehow, by chance, it replicated itself. And somehow this original life form went on to evolve into you and me. If one does not believe in a God who created life, this is the *only* other alternative.

Well, you could say life came from another planet, but then you are still left with explaining how life started there. And unless you believe that all the animals that are alive on earth today came from another planet, you are still left with the belief that life evolved into different organisms. If life were to evolve from simple to complex, it would take a *lot of time*. There is no way around it. By eliminating a Creator God from the picture, one is forced to accept a model based on a very, very long period of time. I do not believe that inanimate atoms could ever result in the formation of a "simple life form" and evolve into a human being no matter how long the time period. Also, the odds against evolution are compounded when you consider that this "simple life form" has to start replicating right away before it dies. And for the "higher" animals, both male and female must evolve simultaneously in order to have offspring.

There are Christians who accept the theory of evolution and try to make the Bible harmonize with the required long time period. This is called theistic evolution. In high school I was given the opportunity to believe in theistic evolution. Father Sirfranco, who taught both biology and religion classes, told the class that you could take the creation account in Genesis literally or you could believe in evolution as long as you believe that at some point in the evolutionary process God introduced a soul. I can remember thinking, *Well which way was it? They both can't be true.*

The fossil record itself provides evidence against evolution. If life started by itself and gradually evolved into other life forms, we would expect to find very few life forms at the bottom of the geologic column and more life forms higher up in the column. However, at the bottom of the column is such a vast number of different life forms that it is known as the Cambrian "explosion."

If "simple" life forms gradually changed into more complex life forms, we would expect to find "transitional" forms in the fossil record, but we do not. What we find is what we would expect when flood waters rose higher and higher, eventually covering all the land. We would expect to find bottom-dwelling marine life at the bottom of the geologic column, then marine fishes and other marine vertebrates, followed by amphibians, reptiles, and finally birds and mammals. Whitcomb and

Morris (1961) provided the reasoning for this order: 1) increasing mobility and therefore increasing ability to postpone inundation; 2) decreasing density and other hydrodynamic factors tending to promote earlier and deeper sedimentation; and 3) increasing elevation of habitat and therefore time required for the flood to attain stages to overtake them.[4]

The best reason for ruling out theistic evolution as the means which God used to create man is that it requires death! God would never use death to create man! Death is an enemy and the day is coming when it will be swallowed up in victory! (1 Corinthians 15:26, 54, 55).

I should make it clear that I do believe in natural selection, also referred to as micro-evolution. We can observe that. The Galapagos finches and the peppered moth are good examples, but natural selection is based on the environment favoring certain genetic strains. The genetic information is already there. Animals best adapted to survive in a certain environment pass on their genes to their progeny. Using micro-evolution as proof for macro-evolution, which requires entirely new genes, is completely unfounded.

Another reason that there are not more scientists taking a stand for a Creator God and against evolution is that it would cost them their jobs. It has happened more times than you know. Ask David Coppedge who was fired from NASA's Jet Propulsion Laboratory for sharing Intelligent Design DVDs with coworkers.[5] Or better yet, read Dr. Jerry Bergman's *Censoring the Darwin Skeptics* in which he documents over 100 cases (60 of whom were PhDs) of discrimination handed out to individuals who dared to challenge evolutionary concepts in schools and scientific institutions.[6]

It makes me laugh as well as feel sad when I hear on the news that we are sending a space craft to some other planet to get clues that will help us understand how life began on earth. We could save a lot of money by reading the first verse in the Bible: "In the beginning God created the heavens and the earth" (Genesis 1:1). Somehow, some people have felt that anything having to do with religion is not scientific. But if religion has the true answer about the origin of life and you eliminate it because it is religious, it leaves you with nothing but false answers. The apostle

Paul warned us about false science: "O Timothy, keep that which is committed to thy trust, avoiding profane and vain babblings, and oppositions of science falsely so called" (1 Timothy 6:20, KJV).

Without the Bible, all we would know about life is what we observe. People are born, live for a while, and die; what happens after that is speculation. The Bible reveals the truth about life on earth. The Bible tells us:

- God created all life on earth in the first week of earth's history (Genesis 1).
- Things were very good until Adam and Eve, our great, great...great grandparents were deceived into believing the serpent (Satan) rather than trusting God (Genesis 3; Revelation 12:9).
- Things drastically deteriorated after that with death, suffering, thorns, thistles, and labor pains becoming part of life on earth (Genesis 3 and 4).
- God put a restoration plan into action with the Creator Himself taking on human nature while keeping His divine nature (Matthew 1 and 2; Luke 2).
- Jesus lived a perfect life, and then paid the death penalty for our disobedience (Matthew, Mark, Luke, and John).
- After three days in the grave, Jesus rose from the dead (Matthew 28; Mark 16; Luke 24; John 20).
- God accepts and forgives anyone who is truly sorry for his sins and asks for forgiveness (1 John 1:9).
- God makes repentant sinners new creations who live their lives trusting in Jesus (2 Corinthians 5:17).
- God gives eternal life to all those trusting in Jesus (1 Thessalonians 4:16).
- God will remake the earth where once again everything will be very good (Revelation 21 and 22).
- God will relocate His throne to the earth where we can talk with Him face to face (Revelation 21 and 22).

- God promises us that sin will never happen again (Nahum 1:9).

Without the Bible, we would have no way of knowing all of this. We would only know what we observe. As scientists, we study nature and understand how the hydrologic cycle works and how the nutrient cycle works. We describe photosynthesis and the Krebs cycle, but without the Bible we do not know the true meaning of life. We do not know that the nature we observe is not normal, that thorns and thistles, labor pains, suffering, and death are not the true norm. True nature is temporarily on hold until sin is eradicated. The true norm, life on earth as it was intended to be, will be restored and when it is, it will be permanent! (Nahum 1:9). What a difference understanding these things has made in my life and in the lives of millions of other people.

Understanding the Bible has given me hope in a world that seems to be getting worse every day, where mass shootings are getting to be common place, natural disasters are becoming more intense and more frequent, and the growing national debt in the United States is like a sleeping time bomb. Truly, the "earth is growing old like a garment" (Isaiah 1:6).

When I began reading the Bible I did not automatically assume that it was true. But by the time I finished, I was convinced. The Bible has so many prophecies, including time prophecies written hundreds and thousands of years in advance that were fulfilled exactly as written (more about this in Chapter 27 and Appendix B). Every year, there is more archeological evidence supporting the Bible. But the greatest evidence of the veracity of the Bible is in the thousands of lives that have been changed for the better. To hear some true accounts of changed lives, listen to the radio program Unshackled every night at 9:00 PM Pacific Time. If you live in north Western Washington, tune your radio to 91.1 FM. Otherwise, find it at radioofhope.org/listen.

The greatest evidence for the veracity of the Old Testament comes from Jesus. Jesus believed it was true. He spoke of Noah, Jonah, Daniel, and Moses; He quoted from the Ten Commandments. He constantly prefaced His remarks with "It is written." Speaking of the Old

Testament, Jesus said, "These are they which testify of me" (John 5:39). In His prayer for His disciples just before He was crucified, He prayed to His Father, "Sanctify them by Your truth. Your word is truth" (John 17:17).

The Dead Sea Scrolls, dated between 150 BC and AD 70, give evidence to the accuracy of the Old Testament that we have today. Fragments of every book in the Old Testament were found except the book of Esther. Differences between the Dead Sea Scrolls and today's Old Testament amount to less than 5 percent and most of these differences were in spelling and do not change the meaning.

The quiet time I experienced at the fish hatchery—reading and praying—was just what I needed at this time in my life when my heart was open to God's word. The Bible says, "You will find Him if you seek Him with all your heart and with all your soul" (Deuteronomy 4:29). It took me about one year to finish reading the Bible. At the end of the year on April 14, 1984, on my fortieth birthday, I was baptized and became a member of the Port Townsend Seventh-day Adventist Church.

1. Clark, H. W. 1968. *Fossils, Flood, and Fire.* Outdoor Pictures.

2. Whitcomb, J. C. and H. M. Morris. 1961. *The Genesis Flood.* Presbyterian and Reformed Publishing Company, Phillipsburg, New Jersey.

3. Andre, R. 1951. *Die Flutensagen, etnologisch betrachtet,* cited by Alfred M. Rehwinkel 1957. *The Flood* , Condordia Publishing House, Saint Louis, Missouri, 129.

4. Whitcomb, J. C. and H. M. Morris 1961. *The Genesis Flood,* Presbyterian and Reformed Publishing Company, Phillipsburg, New Jersey, p. 276.

5. https://www.discovery.org/multimedia/?s=Coppedge

6. Bergman, J. 2017. *Censoring the Darwin Skeptics.* Leafcutter Press. https://www.amazon.com/Censoring-Darwin-Skeptics-Eliminating-Dissidents/dp/0981873421

Chapter 12

The Sabbath—Sign of God's Creative Power

"Remember the Sabbath day, to keep it holy." - Exodus 20:8

Accepting the Bible as the word of God has resulted in some changes in my life. One big change was accepting the Sabbath, the seventh day of the week (Saturday), as a day of rest. I learned that there is more to it than merely going to church on a different day. In my early days as a youth, after attending church, I changed my clothes and treated Sunday as I would any other day—playing sports, fishing, working, etc. I did not see it as a 24-hour day of rest, a day to spend some extra time with God in addition to worshiping at church with fellow believers. In this busy, hectic life it is nice to have one day of quiet time to spend with God and not feeling guilty about the grass needing mowing, the house needing painting, the car needing fixing, and all the other things demanding one's time. And in ceasing work for a full day, I am worshiping God. Obedience to God's commandments is the highest form of worship.

I have experienced another big difference between the Sabbath and Sunday. I never associated Sunday with creation. In the first two chapters of the Bible, it tells us that God created everything in six days, that He rested on the seventh-day, and that He blessed the seventh-day and sanctified it (Genesis 2:2). If the Sabbath had been kept by everyone from that first week, I doubt there would be atheists and evolutionists today.

Furthermore, the Sabbath is a weekly reminder of God's creative power. God made everything—except Adam and Eve— out of *nothing*. "He spoke, and it was done; He commanded, and it stood fast" (Psalm 33:9). Now that is power! It is God's same creative power that restores us to His image. The Sabbath is a sign between us and God by which we know that it is God who sanctifies us (Ezekiel 20:12).

The Sabbath is the seal of God. It is the only one of the ten commandments that identifies God by name—"The LORD your God"; gives His jurisdiction—"the heavens and the earth, the sea, and all that is in them"; and states the basis of His authority— "in six days the LORD made the heavens and the earth, the sea, and all that is in them."

God desires a relationship with us, and a relationship requires time. That's why He told us to refrain from work on the Sabbath—so we could spend some extra time with Him and with each other. The Sabbath lasts for 24 hours. It starts at sundown Friday and ends at sundown Saturday (Leviticus 23:5, 32; Mark 1:32). That keeping the Sabbath is important can be seen by the fact that it is one of the Ten Commandments that God wrote in stone with His own finger and spoke out loud at Mount Sinai (Exodus 20:1; 24:12).

So why do most Christians worship on Sunday? The reason generally given is that Jesus rose from the dead on Sunday, the first day of the week. That is true, but nowhere in the Bible does God say that he sanctified the first day of the week and tell us not to work on it as He did the seventh day. That it is a particular seventh day and not any seventh day can be seen by the definite article "the" Sabbath as opposed to the indefinite article "a" Sabbath. It is the day that Jesus and his disciples kept holy. That it was in effect before God wrote it on stone can be seen in Exodus 16 when God rebuked the Israelites for collecting manna on the Sabbath. The Bible tells us that we will be keeping the Sabbath on the New Earth (Isaiah 66:23).

Sunday-keeping in the Christian Church is a very old tradition, going back to at least the fourth century when the Roman Emperor Constantine issued a decree that Sunday be a day of rest in honor of the "venerable day of the sun." But a tradition is still a tradition and when it goes against a commandment of God, it is best to obey God's commandment. Jesus warned us about keeping a tradition instead of obeying a commandment (Mark 7:9–13). Daniel prophesied that someone would try to change God's law (Daniel 7:25).

I have studied this subject thoroughly and believe the final test before Jesus returns will be over the day of rest—resting on a day based on a commandment of God versus on a tradition of man. Revelation 14:12 clearly tells us that in the last days His saints will be keeping His commandments. Genuine faith is not only believing what God says but acting on it. That is what the disciple James meant when he said, "faith by itself, if it does not have works, is dead" (James 2:17). Jesus obeyed his Father's commands and His people will also.

I want to make it clear that it is not resting on God's true Sabbath day that saves us. It is the One we worship who saves us. His name is Jesus. "Nor is there salvation in any other, for there is no other name under heaven given among men by which we must be saved" (Acts 4:12). We keep the seventh-day Sabbath holy because we love Jesus. Jesus said, "If you love Me, keep My commandments" (John 14:15).

I love my Lord Jesus and I hope you love Him too. I hope you love Him enough to obey all His commandments.

Chapter 13
Modern Day Prophet

for prophecy never came by the will of man, but holy men of God spoke as they were moved by the Holy Spirit. - 2 Peter 1:21

On one of my visits to the church in White Salmon while staying at the hatchery, I was invited to someone's home for lunch after the worship service. While there I was given the book *Ellen G. White, Prophet of Destiny* by Rene Noorbergen.[1] Seventh-day Adventists believe that Ellen White was a modern-day prophet. I have to say that when I first heard of her I was skeptical. My first thought was that a modern-day prophet would be well known and I had never heard of her, not even when I lived in her home state of Maine. However, the more I investigated her, the more I became convinced that she truly was a prophet of God and more than a prophet, as she referred to herself as God's messenger. She was given visions of past as well as of future events. In her own words:

> As inquiries are frequently made as to my state in vision, and after I come out, I would say that when the Lord sees fit to give a vision, I am taken into the presence of Jesus and angels, and am entirely lost to earthly things. I can see no farther than the angel directs me. My attention is often directed to scenes transpiring upon earth. At times I am carried far ahead into the future and shown what is to take place. Then again I am shown things as they have occurred in the past.[2]

Now I will ask you a question, "Which is more dangerous, to believe a false prophet or not to believe a true prophet?" I think that one is just as bad as the other. God's people were led astray by false prophets in the past (Jeremiah 5:31; Ezekiel 22:8) and Jesus warned us about false prophets coming in His name in the future (Matthew 7:15; 24:11, 24).

However, to disregard the words spoken by true prophets also leads to catastrophe. For example, God's people were made captives in Babylon because they did not listen to His prophets. Daniel acknowledged this in his fervent prayer as the reason they were in Babylon: "Neither have we heeded Your servants the prophets, who spoke in Your name" (Daniel 9:6).

This is particularly significant because some of God's people are in spiritual Babylon today and God is calling them out lest they receive the seven last plagues: "Come out of her [Babylon], my people, lest you share in her sins, and lest you receive of her plagues" (Revelation 18:4). The Bible does say that there will be prophets in the last days (Joel 2:28).

I urge you to prayerfully investigate Ellen White for yourself comparing her words to the words of the Bible, the standard of truth. I have never found anything she has written to disagree with the Bible, but you will find some things described in more detail. For instance, if you really want to find out how horrendous it was on earth during the flood of Noah's day, when Satan feared for his life, read *Patriarchs and Prophets*, pages 90–110.[3]

I have been blessed tremendously by the writings of Ellen White. Her writings have illuminated the words of the Bible and given me a better understanding. Ellen White always lifted up the Bible higher than her own words. She referred to the Bible as the "greater light" and her words as the "lesser light." In her words:

> The Lord has sent His people much instruction, line upon line, precept upon precept, here a little, and there a little. Little heed is given to the Bible, and the Lord has given a lesser light to lead men and women to the greater light. Oh, how much good would be accomplished if the books containing this light were read with a determination to carry out the principles they contain! There would be a thousandfold greater vigilance, a

thousandfold more self-denial and resolute effort. And many more would now be rejoicing in the light of present truth.[4]

Ellen White was a prolific writer and wrote many books, articles, and letters. Of all that she wrote, the book that that she herself said was the most important is *The Great Controversy*.[5] Satan tried to take Ellen White's life as she began to write this book. She only had enough strength to write one page the first day and gradually she was able to write more as her strength increased.

Satan does not want you to read The Great Controversy because it plainly reveals what will soon take place in the closing scenes of earth's history and it reveals his last deceptions. In my life's time I have witnessed the "deadly wound" of the sea beast, spoken of in Revelation, being healed (Revelation 13:1-3). In *The Great Controversy* you will learn who the "sea beast" is and what the dreaded "mark of the beast" is (Revelation 13:17). It is not my intention to repeat everything written in *The Great Controversy. I urge you to obtain a copy and prayerfully read it!*

1. Noorbergen, R. 1972. *Ellen G. White: Prophet of Destiny*. Keats Publishing, Inc, New Canaan, Connecticut.

2. *Selected Messages From the Writings of Ellen G. White*, Book One, 1958, Review and Herald Publishing Association, Washington, DC.

3. White, E. G. 1958. *Patriarchs and Prophets*. Review and Herald Publishing Association, Mountain View, California, 13.

4. White, E. G. 1995. *Ye Shall Receive Power*. Review and Herald Publishing Association, Hagerstown, Maryland, 232.

5. White, E. G. 1911. *The Great Controversy*. Review and Herald Publishing Association, Mountain View, California.

Chapter 14
Transferred to Pennsylvania

Let him who stole steal no longer, but rather let him labor, working with his hands what is good, that he may have something to give him who has need. - Ephesians 4:28

Priorities and funding constantly change in the federal government and I was receiving warnings that funding for my position was about to run out, so I began searching the "green sheets" for a good place to go. I came close to working for the Bureau of Indian Affairs (BIA) in Metlakatla, Alaska, but at the last minute the funding fell through. My next choice was Wellsboro, Pennsylvania. Wellsboro is in north central Pennsylvania and is about fifteen miles south of the New York border. One benefit of working there was that it was about half way between Linda's family near Buffalo, New York and my brother Chris' family in Paramus, New Jersey. Another good point was that north central Pennsylvania is fairly rural and there was plenty of state land and farm land to hunt and fish on. Besides those advantages, I would be involved with acid rain research and the work interested me.

In July 1984, three months after I was baptized, we moved to Wellsboro. The Fish and Wildlife Service paid for the move. Movers loaded all our possessions except our Old Town canoe into a moving van. We took the canoe on top of our 1969 microbus, which Linda had purchased new before moving to Washington. We turned the trip into a vacation and stopped at scenic places along the way. In Grand Teton National Park we took a canoe paddle across crystal clear Jenny Lake.

In those days I grew a beard during the cool months and shaved it off when it warmed up. On our trip east it warmed up in Wyoming. When two-year-old Heather first saw me with a shaven face, she was not too sure who I was. But in a little while she got used to me.

Linda has always been one for taking the "back roads." I call her "back roads Linda." Naturally, we avoided the Interstate and stayed on the back roads all the way to Pennsylvania. However, when Linda took a wrong turn, she really got onto a back road. She described it as a narrow, winding, rocky road with a drop-off along the edge. The road's steepness required her shifting down to first gear. We were carrying a keg of reloading powder and Linda was worrying about it exploding should we go off the edge of the road. Eventually, the road came out to a less treacherous back road and we continued heading east. What was I doing during this hair-raising part of the trip? Sleeping, of course!

After about a week of driving, we arrived at our destination and began looking for a temporary place to stay while looking for a house to rent. We found a little cabin in a resort called Frome Acres. The cabin turned out to be our home for the next three months as we had a difficult time finding a house to rent. In the mean time there were lots of cottontail rabbits in the yard to help keep Dawn, Heather, and Jake occupied and Pine Creek was right out in back. Pine Creek flows through a gorge with high canyon walls. It is called the Grand Canyon of Pennsylvania.

Jeanie of Frome Acres operated a rafting business on Pine Creek. She invited us to join her group of rafters on one of her trips. The group turned out to be teenage boys. They were in several rafts and immediately started having fun splashing each other. The water was cold and I was thinking, *they are going to be shivering before too long.* As it turned out, they did more than shiver and started suffering the effects of hypothermia. We watched one raft pull into shore. Several boys jumped out, and started walking down a railroad track paralleling the river. We paddled to shore and I ran after them. They did not know where they were going or what they were doing. I got them to return to our canoe and we gave them dry clothes from our "dump bags" to put on. Eventually, we all made it safely to the take out.

After much searching we found a two-story house to rent next to a mobile home court in Niles Valley, a little community outside of Wellsboro. We did not realize it until later, but the country road that the house was on was a major coal route and convoys of coal trucks constantly rumbled by.

It did not take Linda long to start a garden. The hot summer days were perfect for growing tomatoes and melons. One day we were standing by the garden talking to a neighbor. The conversation turned to the cantaloupes growing there—whether they were ripe or not. As we were talking, I looked down to see Jake chewing away on one. I cut off a piece and tried it. It was ripe!

Another day, Linda and Nicholas, a little boy from the trailer court, were removing Japanese beetle larvae from the garden. While Linda was concentrating on the larvae, Nicholas said, "There's a bear over there."

"There are no bears around here," Linda replied. But looking through some rose bushes, Linda could see something large and black. She immediately thought of some black angus cattle that were pastured not far away and surmised that one must have gotten out. Not wanting it to get on the road, Linda started circling around to put herself between the animal and the road. It was then that she saw it clearly. Nicholas was right. It was a bear and a good size bear at that. The bear crossed the road, stepped over a fence, and headed out across the field.

The closest I have ever come to a tornado occurred while living in Pennsylvania. I noticed the air taking on a greenish color. Soon after that, cars began backing up on the road in front of the house. A tornado had touched down about a mile away. It damaged several houses and uprooted a number of trees.

It was a short commute from Niles Valley to the Fish and Wildlife facility in Asaph. The large building, containing row after row of laboratory benches, was a whole lot different from the converted light keeper's house back in Washington.

Our acid rain research site was in the Pocono Mountains, 150 miles to the east. On a large tract of pristine land, owned by the Blooming Grove Hunting and Fishing Club, flowed two streams, which joined one another. Water in one stream was stained brown with tannin; the other stream ran clear. The objective of the study was to compare the ecology of the two streams before and after treating each with limestone.

After measuring the pH in these streams and finding it less than 5.0 (highly acidic) in each, I became a believer in acid rain. Mudminnows, which are tolerant of acidic water, and a single American eel were the only fish we saw in these streams. Pennsylvania is downwind from a lot of sulfur dioxide-producing smoke stacks in the Ohio Valley, and Pennsylvania itself is a major producer of this gas which turns into sulfuric acid when combined with rain. Nitrogen oxides, precursors of nitric acid, from automobile exhausts added to the acidity of the rainfall.

In Pennsylvania we were within a day's drive of the camp and went as often as we could. Those three years in Pennsylvania would be the last years that I would be able to enjoy the camp. However, I had one thing on my mind that I had to do at the camp that was not enjoyable at all. When I had worked for General Electric at the firing range, I had stolen an ammo can full of 7.62 mm casings, which were still at the camp. As a newly baptized Christian, I knew I had to return them. Not knowing what they would do, I made the seventy-mile drive to the firing range and told the security guard why I was there. He brought me to the manager, and I told him what I had done. Thankfully, he did not press charges and I drove back with a lighter heart and praising God.

Chapter 15
Change in Diet

"These you may eat of all that are in the water: whatever in the water has fins and scales, whether in the seas or in the rivers—that you may eat. But all in the seas or in the rivers that do not have fins and scales, all that move in the water or any living thing which is in the water, they are an abomination to you." - Leviticus 11:9, 10

Before I was baptized, I learned that God did not put everything on the food menu. He differentiated between clean and unclean animals as described in Deuteronomy 14. Only clean animals are to be eaten. Clean animals are those that have split hooves and chewed a cud. Clean fish are those with both scales and fins. Clean birds are distinguished from unclean birds by listing the unclean ones which included eagles, vultures, and ravens. I looked through the Bible for the reason for not having the unclean animals on the food list but could not find any. However, it appears that clean animals forage on vegetation whereas unclean animals are scavengers or predators.

I do not believe God made up an arbitrary list. I believe He separated the unclean from the clean because He loves us and did not want us eating anything unhealthy. If certain animals were not healthy in the past, they are not healthy now. The Bible says that "your body is the temple of the Holy Spirit who is in you, whom you have from God, and you are not your own" (1 Corinthians 6:19) and "whether you eat or drink or whatever you do, do all to the Glory of God" (1 Corinthians 10:31).

The Bible says that faith is the victory that overcomes the world (1

John 5:4) and without faith it is impossible to please God (Hebrews 11:6). Another way of saying I have *faith in God* is to say I *believe God* or I *trust God*. I know God loves me and everything God says to do or not to do is for my good. If we understood everything, there would be no room for faith. I have no doubt that a lot of disease and suffering would be avoided by following God's counsel on diet. There is much truth in the saying: *An ounce of prevention is worth a pound of cure*.

My work for the Conservation District has given me plenty of reason for not eating shellfish, which have neither scales nor fins. My work involves monitoring fecal coliform bacteria in streams flowing into Puget Sound. Fecal coliform bacteria originate in the digestive tract of all warm-blooded animals, including humans, and are released into the environment by excretion. They serve as indicators of potential disease-causing bacteria and viruses released with them. Bacterial pathogens of greatest concern are *Vibrio, Salmonella, Shigella, Escherichia, Listeria, Yersinea, Campylobacter*, and *Leptospira*. [1,2] Viruses include hepatitis A, hepatitis E, poliovirus, NLVs (Norwalk-like viruses), SRSVs (small round structured viruses), and caliciviruses.[2]

Shellfish, including oysters, clams, mussels, cockles, and scallops are filter-feeders. They feed on phytoplankton and can bioaccumulate any pathogens present in the surrounding water. Diarrhea, caused by gastroenteritis, is the most common symptom of consuming infected shellfish. In 1988, 290,000 people in Shanghai became sick and 47 people died from eating hepatitis A-contaminated clams. Other large outbreaks of bivalve-associated infections involving greater than 800 people occurred in Australia in 1979, the United States in 1986, and Japan in 1991. Since 1970, global consumption of shellfish has increased considerably, and with it, reports of outbreaks of infection.[2]

The Center for Disease Control and Prevention reported that about 80,000 people are infected with *Vibrio* and 100 people die from it in the United States every year. Most of the illnesses are from eating raw or undercooked oysters, but other shellfish, such as clams and mussels, also infect people. *Vibrio parahaemolyticus*, the most common agent of vibriosis, causes diarrhea and vomiting. However, *Vibrio vulnificus*, a rarer species, can make people extremely sick and can result in bloodstream infections, severe blistering skin lesions, and limb amputations. As many as one in five infected people die from it.[3]

Besides bacteria and viruses, shellfish may also bioaccumulate toxic phytoplankton. These algae can increase exponentially forming blooms commonly called "red tide," but formally known as harmful algal blooms or HABs. In recent decades, HABs have increased dramatically in intensity and frequency in coastal regions around the world.[4] Speaking about HABs in Puget Sound, shellfish biologist Kart Mueller said, "In recent years, warming water temperatures have contributed to frequent HABs in the nearshore areas of the Lummi Nation, which is consistent with current climate change predictions."[5]

Currently, about 100 algal species are known to produce toxins that cause sickness or death.[6] Four of the most common HAB-related illnesses from shellfish consumption are Paralytic Shellfish Poisoning (PSP), Neurotoxin Shellfish Poisoning (NSP), Diarrheic Shellfish Poisoning (DSP), and Amnesic Shellfish Poisoning (ASP). Unlike harmful bacteria and viruses, toxins from phytoplankton are not destroyed by cooking.

The most risky regions for Paralytic Shellfish Poisoning are cold-water coasts. Initial symptoms of mild PSP are numbness or tingling around the mouth and lips within ten minutes to two hours of shellfish consumption. I experienced this soon after eating a bowl of chowder containing mussels from Puget Sound. Within a short time after eating the chowder, my lips began to tingle. In more severe cases, the numbness and tingling spread to the neck and face and may be accompanied by headache, abdominal pain, nausea, vomiting, diarrhea, and a wide range of neurological symptoms. These neurological symptoms may include weakness, dizziness, double vision, and loss of coordination. In the most severe cases, symptoms rapidly progress to severe respiratory problems and sometimes death.[7]

The most risky region for Neurotoxin Shellfish Poisoning is the Gulf of Mexico, especially along the west coast of Florida. Symptom onset ranges from a few minutes to eighteen hours; three to four hours is most common. Symptoms include both gastrointestinal and neurological problems. The most frequently reported symptoms are nausea, vomiting, abdominal pain, and diarrhea. Neurological symptoms include tingling of the mouth, lips, and tongue, partial limb paralysis, slurred speech, dizziness, and a general loss of coordination.[7]

Diarrheic Shellfish Poisoning has occurred in the United States,[8] Japan, Europe, Canada, New Zealand, United Kingdom, and South America. Symptom onset typically occurs within 30 minutes to 4 hours after shellfish consumption. The main symptom is incapacitating diarrhea, followed by nausea, vomiting, and abdominal cramps. Although DSP poisoning is traditionally believed to result in full recovery, preliminary data raises the possibility that DSP toxins may be associated with more significant medical problems over time.[7]

Where I live in Washington State, Amnesic Shellfish Poisoning is more commonly referred to as Domoic Acid, the toxin in the phytoplankton. The potential risk of ASP to human health was first discovered in 1987 in Montreal, Canada. Persons who ate affected blue mussels harvested from the Prince Edward Island region suffered serious medical illnesses including death. Survivors were left with a permanent and profound memory disorder.[7]

Within the past twenty years, Domoic Acid levels have been significantly elevated along the Pacific Coast and razor clams are particularly affected. A recent study focused on 513 Native American adult men and women who ate fifteen or more razor clams per month from the Pacific Coast over a four-year period. The group had isolated declines in some measures of memory, although the relatively lower memory scores were still within normal limits. The authors concluded that there is a possible association between memory function and long-term, low-level exposure to Domoic Acid through heavy razor clam consumption.[7]

Based on a follow-up study on a cross section of sixty of the men and women who were exposed to low levels of Domoic Acid from eating razor clams the previous week and during the past year, the researchers concluded that Native Americans who eat a lot of razor clams with presumably safe levels of Domoic Acid are at risk for clinically significant memory problems. The researchers said that there is now in place public health outreach to minimize repetitive exposures.[9] Razor clams hold the toxin up to one year in the natural environment and up to several years after being processed, canned, or frozen.[7]

From 1973 to 2006, there were 2,810 illnesses reported in the United States due to shellfish contaminated with bacteria or viruses.[10] This number is an under representation because the number of illnesses per year increased substantially after 1998 when surveillance increased. Without laboratory analysis, one cannot tell if a clam, oyster, or other shellfish contains harmful bacteria, viruses, or toxins. Given the risk of eating contaminated shellfish, it seems wise to follow God's counsel (Leviticus 11:9, 10) and avoid them.

1. Lilja, J. and S. Glasoe. 1993. Uses and limitations of coliform indicators in shellfish sanitation programs. *Puget Sound Notes* 30:4–6.

2. Potasman, I., A. Paz, and M. Odeh. 2002. Infectious outbreaks associated with bivalve shellfish consumption: A worldwide perspective. *Clinical Infectious Diseases* 35(8):921–928. https://doi.org/10.1086/342330.

3. www.cdc.gov/features/vibrio-raw-oysters/index.html

4. Glibert, P.M., D.M. Anderson, P. Gentien, E. Granéli, and K.G. Sellner. 2005. The global, complex phenomena of harmful algal blooms. *Oceanography* 18(2):136–147. https://doi.org/10.5670/oceanog.2005.49.

5. Neumeyer, K. 2019. Testing shellfish for biotoxins. Northwest Treaty Tribes, Olympia, Washington, Summer 2019.

6. Farabegoli, F., L. Blanco, L. P. Roddriguez, J. M. Vieites, and A. G. Cabado. 2018. Phycotoxins in marine shellfish: origin, occurrence and effects on humans. *Marine Drugs* 16(6):188. doi:10.3390/md16060188.

7. Grattan, L. M., S. Holobaugh, and J. G. Morris, Jr. Harmful algal blooms and public health. *Harmful Algae* 57(B):2–8.

8. Lloyd, J. K., J. S. Duchin, J. Borchert, H. F. Quintana, and A. Robertson. 2013. Diarrhetic shellfish poisoning, Washington, USA, 2011. *Emerging Infectious Diseases* 19(8):1314–1316.

9. Grattan, L. M., C. J. Boushey, Y. Liang, K. A. Lefebvre, L. J. Castellon, K. A. Roberts, A. C. Toben, and J. G. Morris. 2018.

Repeated dietary exposure to low levels of Domoic acid and problems with everyday memory: Research to public health outreach. *Toxins* 10(3):103.

10. Iwamoto, M., T. Ayers, B. E. Mahon, and D. L. Swerdlow. 2010. Epidemiology of seafood-associated infections in the United States. *Clinical Microbiology Reviews* 23(2):399-411.

Chapter 16
More Changes in Diet and a Big Change in Lifestyle

Therefore, whether you eat or drink, or whatever you do, do all to the glory of God. - 1 Corinthians 10:31

While in Pennsylvania something happened to me that I would never have thought possible. I became a vegetarian! When I was baptized, I had no intention of becoming a vegetarian, but I had not counted on the promptings of the Holy Spirit.

The original diet before sin entered the world was a vegetarian diet for both man and animals. In Genesis 1:29, 30, we read: "And God said, 'See, I have given you every herb that yields seed which is on the face of all the earth, and every tree whose fruit yields seed; to you it shall be for food. Also, to every beast of the earth, to every bird of the air, and to everything that creeps on the earth, in which there is life, I have given every green herb for food'; and it was so." A diet of meat requires death. Had Adam and Eve not sinned there would be no death on planet earth, not even in the animal kingdom. If this seems doubtful to you, consider the way it will be on the New Earth one day when sin has been eradicated forever. Isaiah prophesied about the animals on the New Earth: "the wolf and the lamb shall feed together, and the lion shall eat straw like the ox" (Isaiah 65:25).

In my early days of reading the Bible I was a little doubtful when I first read about "the lion eating straw like the ox." It seemed like those huge canine teeth were designed for capturing and devouring prey. Then

God swept away my doubt with a true story about a vegetarian lioness named Little Tyke.[1] Little Tyke was mauled by its mother soon after its birth in a zoo in Washington State. The little cub, with a broken leg, was given into the care of a couple who had a ranch on the Green River. When it was weaned from bottled milk, they gave it meat to eat, but Little Tyke refused to eat it. However, Little Tyke readily ate the diet the couple prepared for it: a variety of grains, eggs, and milk, which Little Tyke supplemented by eating tall grass in the field. Little Tyke was friendly to the other animals on the farm as well as to people and was in parades and on television. She died of pneumonia at the age of nine. It is a touching story and gives us a preview of how wonderful it will be on the New Earth when men and animals all get along together. I long for that day! I no longer have any doubts about what the Bible says. If the Bible says it, I believe it!

The report I had written on sturgeon and the high levels of PCBs which they contain started me thinking about how contaminated fish are. Then I read Ellen White's book, *The Ministry of Healing*.[2] Published in 1905, this book was ahead of its time concerning contaminants in fish. In the book Ellen wrote a chapter titled *Flesh as Food,* and in this chapter she wrote one paragraph on fish:

> In many places fish become so *contaminated* by the filth on which they feed as to be a cause of disease. This is especially the case where the fish come in contact with the sewage of large cities. The fish that are fed on the contents of the drains may pass into distant waters and may be caught where the water is pure and fresh. Thus when used as food they bring disease and death on those who do not suspect the danger (emphasis mine).

Since the industrial revolution of the 1800s, a vast array of chemicals has been manufactured and released into the environment. Our lakes and rivers have become an alphabet soup of chemicals—DDT, DDE, DDD, PFOA, PFOS, PCBs, PBDEs, PFCs, PAHs, etc. Many of these chemicals bioaccumulate in fish and cause cancer, birth defects, behavioral changes, and cognitive disabilities. The following is an account of two of the most studied contaminants: mercury and polychlorinated biphenyls (PCBs).

Mercury

Mercury is an element, occurring naturally in the environment. Bacteria soon convert elemental mercury to methylmercury, the form that bioaccumulates in the food chain. Mercury enters the atmosphere from erupting volcanoes and it is spread by atmospheric winds.[3, 4] Mercury occurs in trace amounts in coal. When coal is burned to produce electricity, it escapes into the atmosphere and can come down thousands of miles from its source. The United States is downwind from China and undoubtedly receives atmospheric mercury from China's coal-burning power plants. In 2011, China consumed 3.6 billion tons of coal.[5] In the past 150 years, human activities are believed to have increased the mercury concentration three- to five-fold in the atmosphere[6] and three-fold in the upper ocean.[7]

In the United States from 2010 to 2012, 82 percent of population-wide exposure to methylmercury was from the consumption of estuarine and marine seafood with 37 percent of that being from fresh and canned tuna alone.[7.5] Elevated blood mercury levels occurred more commonly among women of childbearing age living in coastal areas of the United States. The highest levels occurred in the Northeast, followed by the South and West; the lowest levels were in the Midwest.[8]

In 2011, more than 16 million lake-acres and one million river-miles were under fish consumption advisories due to mercury contamination; all 50 states had fish consumption advisories due to mercury.[9] Even fish from our pristine National Parks are contaminated with mercury. In a study of 1,400 fish, collected at 86 sites across 21 national parks in the Western United States, 68 percent of the fish sampled exceeded levels recommended by the Great Lakes Advisory Group for unlimited consumption.[3]

Mercury is associated with birth deformities, neuropsychological dysfunctions, diminished IQs, high blood pressure, coronary heart disease, heart attack, and stroke. (See Appendix A for supporting studies.)

PCBs

Polychlorinated biphenyls, commonly known as PCBs, are man-made compounds which were used as heat exchange fluids in transformers, capacitors, and light ballasts as well as in caulking, sealants, and paints from the 1930s to the 1970s. They were banned in the United States in 1979.

PCBs are chlorinated hydrocarbons, a class of chemicals known for their persistence in the environment, their ability to bioaccumulate in the food chain, and their toxicity to animals and humans. The harmful effects of chlorinated hydrocarbons were first brought to the attention of the public in 1962 by scientist Rachel Carson in her famous book *Silent Spring*.[10] In this book she clearly and meticulously laid out the harmful effects of DDT and other chlorinated hydrocarbon pesticides on birds, animals, and humans. She said that pesticides would be more properly termed *biocides* because their effects are rarely limited to the target pests.

PCBs, although designed for a different purpose, have proven to have the same biocide characteristics as DDT and other chlorinated hydrocarbon pesticides. PCBs bioaccumulate in a wide variety of fish and fish-eating birds and animals, including eagles, ospreys, gulls, terns, herons, cormorants, seals, dolphins, whales, bears, mink, and otter.

There are 209 congeners or forms of PCBs, based on the number and placement of chlorine atoms on the biphenyl ring. Each congener has its own toxicity level. The greatest impact of PCBs is on the developing child in the womb and for the next several years after birth. As the fertilized egg multiplies and differentiates into the various body parts, organs, and systems, there is much room for things to go wrong.

It is amazing that the fetus develops perfectly a very high percentage of the time. The psalmist was right when he said, "I will praise You, for I am fearfully and wonderfully made; marvelous are Your works, and that my soul knows very well" (Psalm 138:14).

In 2011, over 6 million lake-acres and over 131 thousand river-miles were under consumption advisories for PCBs.[9] This was an increase of 8,164 lake-acres and an increase of 433 river miles from the previous year. We should understand that most fish species in most of our streams and lakes have never been analyzed for any potential contaminants. Thus advisories increase each year as more fish in more waterbodies are tested.

High doses of PCBs in rice oil have caused acne-like skin eruptions, liver cancer, liver cirrhosis, and enlarged liver. Some babies born to mothers who ate the PCB-contaminated rice oil died from pneumonia, bronchitis, and sepsis (bacterial infection of the blood).

Babies born to mothers who ate PCB-contaminated fish from Lake Michigan were smaller, had abnormally weak reflexes, reduced responsiveness, reduced motor coordination, and reduced muscle tone. At seven months the children exhibited decreased visual recognition and had possible neurological impairment. At four years, they had slower reactions to visual stimuli, more errors and longer times to solve memory tests, diminished attention control and information retention, and possible hyperactivity. At eleven years their IQ scores were inversely correlated to PCB levels in the umbilical cord blood and maternal blood and milk. (See Appendix A for supporting studies.)

Fish Consumption Advisories

Fish consumption advisories generally point out that fish are nutritious and contain omega-3 fatty acids that are good for the heart and brain. The following is taken from the Washington State Department of Health website[11] with slight formatting changes:

> Fish is a low-fat high quality protein. Fish is filled with omega-3 fatty acids and vitamins such as D and B2 (riboflavin). Fish is rich in calcium and phosphorus and a great source of minerals, such as iron, zinc, iodine, magnesium, and potassium. The American Heart Association recommends eating fish at least two times per week as part of a healthy diet. Fish is packed with protein, vitamins, and nutrients that can lower blood pressure and help reduce the risk of a heart attack or stroke. Learn how to properly cook fish and try some healthy recipes. Choose seafood that's low in contaminants and high in health benefits.

Eating fish is an important source of omega-3 fatty acids. These essential nutrients keep our heart and brain healthy. Two omega-3 fatty acids found in fish are EPA (eicosapentaenoic acid) and DHA (docosahexaenoic acid). Our bodies don't produce omega-3 fatty acids so we must get them through the food we eat. Omega-3 fatty acids are found in every kind of fish, but are especially high in fatty fish. Some good choices are salmon, trout, sardines, herring, canned mackerel, canned light tuna, and oysters.

Omega-3 Fatty Acids: help maintain a healthy heart by lowering blood pressure and reducing the risk of sudden death, heart attack, abnormal heart rhythms, and strokes; aid healthy brain function and infant development of vision and nerves during pregnancy; may decrease the risk of depression, ADHD, Alzheimer's disease, dementia, and diabetes; and may prevent inflammation and reduce the risk of arthritis.

Fish is an important cultural icon in Washington State that defines a recreational as well as a spiritual way of life in the Pacific Northwest. Fish is not only an important source of nutrition, the act of catching, preparing, and eating fish are important cultural and family practices as well. To Native American Indian Tribes of Washington, fish, especially salmon, are an integral part of their lives, and serve as a symbol of their prosperity, culture, and heritage.

The problem is that the omega-3 fatty acids reside in the fatty part of the fish, the same place where PCBs and other persistent contaminants reside! The consumer is left with the decision of what kind of fish to eat, where they come from, how many to eat, and how often to eat them. These figures are continually being adjusted as more information becomes available. In 2017, the EPA had this to say regarding consumption advisories:

Some subsistence fishers, tribes, sport fishers and other groups consume large amounts of contaminated fish without health warnings. Although most states and some tribes have fish advisories in place, this information is often confusing, complex and does not effectively reach those segments of the population. Fish advisories differ from state to state, between states and tribes, and across state and tribal borders, which in some cases leads to multiple advisories with conflicting advice for a single waterbody. In addition, although the EPA's Risk Communication Guidance recommends evaluations of fish advisories, we found that less than half of states, and no tribes, have evaluated the effectiveness of their fish advisories.[12]

Endocrine-Disrupting Chemicals

In 1996, the book *Our Stolen Future: Are We Threatening Our Fertility, Intelligence, and Survival? A Scientific Detective Story* by Theo Colborn, Dianne Dumanoski, and John Peterson Myers brought attention to an emerging field of study—endocrine-disrupting chemicals or EDCs.[13] Since then, hundreds of studies on EDCs, including PCBs and mercury, have been shown to affect fish, reptiles, birds, animals, and humans.

Hormones are chemical messengers that travel through the blood to other parts of the body where they communicate and coordinate with other tissues. They are produced by endocrine tissues such as the ovaries, testes, adrenal, pituitary, thyroid, and pancreas. Hormones work with the nervous system, reproductive system, kidneys, gut, liver, and fat to help maintain and control body energy levels, reproduction, growth and development, and internal balance. EDCs can interfere with the body's own hormone signals because of their similar structure.[14]

Development and regulation of the reproductive system is one of the major functions of the endocrine system. Sex determination and development begin early in gestation, with differentiation of the embryonic gonad into either testes or ovaries. For males and females alike, the entire process of reproductive development is exquisitely sensitive to minute changes in levels of sex hormones, particularly during certain critical windows of development.[14]

Fetal development is such a delicately timed and precisely controlled process that there is much opportunity for something to go wrong. Mimicking the body's hormones, EDCs can disrupt differentiation and development in a wide variety of ways: by duplicating, exaggerating, blocking, or altering hormonal responses. Furthermore, fetal and neonatal exposure to low doses of EDCs may not be immediately recognizable, but could alter metabolism, cause infertility, and/or cause cancer later in life.[15]

Of approximately 85,000 known chemical products, about 1,000 are recognized as potential EDCs, a number of which are persistent chlorinated hydrocarbons that bioaccumulate in the aquatic food chain.[16] We now know that EDCs have been responsible for reproductive abnormalities (intersex offspring) and reproductive failures resulting in population declines in a large number of fish species; fish-eating birds: eagles, ospreys, gulls, terns, and cormorants; mammals: mink, otter, and bear; amphibians: frogs and salamanders; and reptiles: alligators and turtles. There is mounting evidence that the increasing trend in breast cancer and prostate cancer[17] and increasing trend in children born with both male and female genitals[18] are caused by EDCs.

Eating fish is not the only way to become contaminated with EDCs, but it is one of them. It is noteworthy that state and federal agencies singularly focus on fish and shellfish in their consumption advisories.

If anyone was qualified to verify that Ellen White's statement that fish are contaminated is true, it was me. I was being convicted by the Holy Spirit to make a change, but a large part of me was saying, "*No!*" Eating three meat-packed meals a day had been my diet for forty years. But it was much more than diet. It was a lifestyle and there was nothing I enjoyed more than fishing and hunting. For six months a battle raged within me. Finally, I surrendered to the Holy Spirit. I gathered up my rifles and shotguns, took them to the sporting goods store in Wellsboro, and sold them all. I thought that life would never be enjoyable after that.

One day it dawned on me that there would be no fishing in Heaven. This thought had no sooner entered my mind when a Bible verse came to me. It was from 1 Corinthians 2:9: "Eye has not seen, nor ear heard, nor have entered into the heart of man the things which God has prepared for those who love Him." It was immediately followed by this thought as if God was speaking to me: *Glenn, if you think you liked fishing, you just wait to see what I have in store for you.* From that day forward, God performed a miracle and took my desire to hunt and fish and eat flesh foods completely away and I have never looked back.

Thankfully, Linda, who does about all the cooking in our home, accommodated me in my diet change. She sometimes reminds me of a comment I made before we were married. We were at Linda's home on Lake Washington and she was stirring a black iron kettle on her stove. I was looking into the kettle to see what was rising to the surface.

After looking for a while and not seeing any meat, I said to her, "You're not one of those vegetarians are you?"

When I had prayed for a wife years before, God who knew us before we were formed in the womb (Jeremiah 1:5; Psalm 139:15, 16), answered my prayer and provided me with a wife who grew up on a vegetable farm. She not only knows how to grow vegetables, she knows how to cook them too!

My Apology

In looking back at my life, fishing was a great blessing as it brought me in close contact with nature, God's second book. (The Bible is His first book.) Fishing has put me in places where I experienced sights that I otherwise would have missed. I remember:

- watching a mother mink leading her family of young right past me as I stood perfectly still along Cold Brook;
- laughing at several young raccoons near the Genesee River as they fell over backward trying to reach blackberries that were a little too far out of reach;
- watching the amazing dippers (water ouzels) walking underwater, searching for macroinvertebrates to eat;
- two kingfishers creating a commotion on a tree limb over Putts Creek. One had eaten a frog, but could not quite swallow it all. The other kingfisher was tugging on the frog's protruding legs and both fell off the limb into the water.

My closest friendships were developed with fishing and hunting companions. Spending all day in a boat or duck blind together, even an introvert like me can't help but do some talking! After spending so much of my life fishing, it's not easy for me to speak against eating fish. I am not against fishing. With catch and release, one may enjoy the benefits of being in nature without the harmful side effects.

So why am I speaking out? Three reasons:

- first, fish were a major part of "my story" about finding God;
- second, sharing what I have learned about contaminants in fish could save someone from developing cancer or save a child from entering the world physically or mentally handicapped;
- third, sharing the truths I have learned could help someone make sense out of what is going on in this crazy world and give a person hope for the future. The New Earth is coming and anyone who trusts in Jesus can be there!

Would I ever eat fish again? Possibly. If I ever find myself in a situation where fish is all that is available, I would eat fish with thankfulness to God. Currently, I have an abundant variety of foods available from the garden and the supermarket.

I recognize that some people live in areas of the world where there are not as many food options and fish is a staple part of the diet.

We have to make wise choices based on what's available. So make the best choices you can.

---

1. Westbeau, G. H. 1956. *Little Tyke*. Pacific Press Publishing Association, Mountain View, California.

2. White, E. G. 1942. *The Ministry of Healing*, Pacific Press Publishing Association, Mountain View, California, 314, 315.

3. Eagles-Smith, C. A., J. J. Willacker, Jr., C. M. Flanagan Pritz 2014. Mercury in Fishes from 21 National Parks in the Western United States—Inter- and Intra-Park Variation in Concentrations and Ecological Risk. Open File Report 2014-1051, U.S. Geological Survey,

Reston, Virginia. https://pubs.usgs.gov/of/2014/1051/pdf/ofr2014-1051.pdf

4. Lamborg, C. H. and nine other authors 2014. A global ocean inventory of anthropogenic mercury based on water column measurements. *Nature* 512:65–68. https://www.researchgate.net/publication/264634183_A_global_ocean_inventory_of_anthropogenic_mercury_based_on_water_column_measurements

5. Zhou, J., Z. Luo, Y. Zhu, and M. Fang 2013. Controlling pollutants in coal-fired power plants in China. In: Mercury emission and its control in Chinese coal-fired plants. *Advanced Topics in Science and Technology in China.* Springer, Berlin, Heidelberg. https://link.springer.com/chapter/10.1007/978-3-642-37874-4_1

6. Juan, S. 2006. The Minamata disaster—50 years on Lessons learned? *The Register* 14 July 2006. https://www.theregister.co.uk/2006/07/14/the_odd_body_minimata_disaster/

7. Harada, M. 1995. Minamata disease: methylmercury poisoning in Japan caused by environmental pollution. *Critical Reviews in Toxicology* 25(1):1–24.

7.5 Sunderland, E. M., M. Li, and K. Bullard. 2018. Decadal changes in the edible supply of seafood and methylmercury exposure in the United States. *Environmental Health Perspectives* 126:017006. https://doi.org/10.1289/EHP2644

8. Mahaffey, K., R. P. Clickner, R. A. Jeffries. 2009. Adult women's blood mercury concentrations vary regionally in the United States: association with patterns of fish consumption (NHANES 1999–2004). *Environmental Health Perspectives* 117(1):47–53.

9. USEPA 2013. 2011 National Listing of Fish Advisories. Report EPA-820-F-13-058. U.S. Environmental Protection Agency, Washington, DC. https://www.epa.gov/sites/production/files/2015-06/documents/technical-factsheet-2011.pdf

10. Carson, R. 1962; anniversary edition, 2002. *Silent Spring.* Houghton Mifflin Company.

11. Anonymous. Not dated. Washington Department of Health. https://www.doh.wa.gov/CommunityandEnvironment/Food/Fish/Healt hBenefits.

12. Butler, K., J. Hamann, J. Ross, and G. Snyder. 2017. EPA needs to provide leadership and better guidance to improve fish advisory risk communications. Report No. 17-P-0174, U.S. Environmental Protection Agency, Office of Inspector General, Washington.

13. Colborn, T, D. Dumanoski, and J. P. Myers. 1996. *Our Stolen Future: Are We Threatening Our Fertility, Intelligence, and Survival?* A Scientific Detective Story, Dutton, Penguin Books, New York, New York.

14. NIEHS. 2010. *Endocrine disruptors.* National Institute of Environmental Sciences, Research Triangle Park, North Carolina. https://www.niehs.nih.gov/health/materials/endocrine_disruptors_508.p df

15. Hood, E. 2005. Are EDCs Blurring issues of gender? *Environmental Health Perspectives* 113 (10):A670–A677. https://www.ncbi.nlm.nih.gov/pmc/articles/PMC1281309/

16. Street, M. E. and 23 coauthors. 2018. Current knowledge on endocrine disrupting chemicals (EDCs) from animal biology to humans, from pregnancy to adulthood: highlights from a national Italian meeting. *International Journal of Molecular Sciences* 19(6):1647. https://www.ncbi.nlm.nih.gov/pmc/articles/PMC6032228/

17. Soto, A. M. and C. Sonnenschein. 2010. Environmental causes of cancer: endocrine disruptors as carcinogens. *Nature Reviews Endocrinology* 2010:6(7):363–370. https://www.ncbi.nlm.nih.gov/pmc/articles/PMC3933258/

18. Rich, L. M. Phipps, S. Tiwari, H. Rudraraju, and P. O. Dokpes. 2016. The Increasing Prevalence in Intersex Variation from Toxicological Dysregulation in Fetal Reproductive Tissue Differentiation and Development by Endocrine-Disrupting Chemicals. *Environmental Health Insights* 10:163–171. https://www.ncbi.nlm.nih.gov/pmc/articles/PMC5017538/

Chapter 17
A Better Lifestyle

I have come that they may have life, and that they may have it more abundantly. - John 10:10

Seventh-day Adventists are a health-conscious group of people. I have already mentioned that Adventists do not partake of unclean fish, birds, or other animals. Although it is not a requirement, many are vegans or vegetarians. Adventists believe in abstaining from, cigarettes, alcohol, caffeinated coffee, tea and soft drinks, and unnecessary drugs. Fruits, grains, nuts, and vegetables make up the basic diet. Fruits, grains, and nuts were the original diet; vegetables were added a little later.

I stopped drinking alcoholic drinks and caffeinated drinks when I was baptized. I have continued to eat a limited amount of milk and eggs. The Bible says that our body is the temple of the Holy Spirit (1 Corinthians 6:19) and that whatever we eat and drink, we do for the glory of God (1 Corinthians 10:31). The healthier we are and the longer we live, the better we can advance the gospel (Matthew 28:18–20) and hasten the coming of Jesus (2 Peter 3:12) and the New Earth. As bad as this world is getting, the sooner the better!

Seventh-day Adventists operate hospitals and health centers throughout the world. People with health issues may stay at Adventist Health Centers to learn new lifestyle habits. Fifty percent of type 2 diabetics who adopt the NEWSTART° lifestyle are off their insulin and medications in as little as 18 days. Fifty percent of the people with high blood pressure have their blood pressure return to normal levels without the need for medication. Eighty percent of people who suffer from diabetic neuropathy are pain free after 18 days. Some participants on the NEWSTART* program have experienced a 40 percent drop in cholesterol by the end of the program.[1]

NEWSTART* (New Start) is an acronym that comprises eight principles for a healthy lifestyle. The eight principles are preventative in nature and follow the adage: *an ounce of prevention is worth a pound of cure.* When I became an Adventist, I put the eight principles into practice and believe I am healthier for it. Here are the eight principles:

N is for Nutrition. Eat a simple diet consisting of a variety of fruits, nuts, whole grains, and vegetables. Avoid refined sugar and saturated fat. Develop a taste for simple foods prepared in a simple manner. Eat at regular times each day and allow 5–6 hours for digestion between meals. Avoid snacking between meals. Breakfast should be the heartiest meal and supper the lightest if eaten at all. It is best not to eat just before going to bed.

A strict vegan should take a vitamin B_{12} supplement. I obtain vitamin B_{12} in a multivitamin when I have rolled oats for breakfast, which is about every day. I supplement the oats with raisins, walnuts, and almond milk. I make several days worth of vitamin-enhanced almond milk by blending almonds and multivitamins in water. Walnuts are a good way to obtain omega-3 fatty acids in place of fish. Other foods high in omega-3 fatty acids are: chia, hemp, flax, and perilla seeds and oils; canola and algal oils; and Brussels sprouts and spinach.

E is for Exercise. Exercise regularly, preferably outdoors. Exercise is one of the best sleeping aids. Try walking, swimming, cycling, jogging, or gardening.

I like to combine exercise with useful work. We heat with wood and I enjoy getting my own firewood. This gives me exercise several ways: cutting the trees down, cutting them up, splitting the rounds, stacking the wood, and finally moving it to the wood stove.

About 30 years ago, Linda gave me a "monster maul" for splitting wood. The steel wedge is welded to a pipe handle for a total weight of twelve pounds. A friend offered me a hydraulic splitter free, but I turned it down because I knew it would rob me of some exercise. For the same reason, I prefer a push lawn mower as opposed to a self-propelled or riding lawn mower. Walking is good exercise!

I confess that I am not as regular with exercising as I should be. When it is not the firewood season, my muscles get soft. Several years ago Linda brought home a stationary bicycle to exercise on, but it ended up being used as a coat rack. Two weeks ago I moved it into a spare bedroom and set up a TV and DVD player so I could watch something as I peddled. Lately, I have been going for 15-minute bike rides in the morning.

Exercise is very important. A person who smokes and exercises is healthier than one who does not smoke or exercise. It is best to exercise *and* not smoke!

W is for Water. Water is the liquid of life. Our body is about 65 percent water. Our blood is 83 percent water. Water is: the body's transport system; the lubricant for movement; a facilitator for digestion; the prime transporter of waste via the kidneys; a body temperature regulator; and the major constituent of blood.

Start the day with one or two glasses of water and drink another five or six glasses at regular intervals throughout the day. The more active you are, the more you perspire and the more water you need. If you are drinking enough, your urine will be pale and approach the color of water.

It is best to drink pure water and not substitute coffee, tea, or soda. Caffeine in these beverages is harmful. Do not wait until you are thirsty to drink. Keep a water bottle handy and drink frequently. I make it a habit never to go by a drinking fountain without getting a drink.

S is for Sunshine. Obtain sufficient sunshine. Sunshine is the source of vitamin D. It is good for our bones as well as for stimulating the production of some hormones such as melatonin, which assists our sleep, and serotonin, which affects our mood. Sunshine can help counteract depression.

Spend some time in the sun without overdoing it and getting sunburned. Morning and late afternoon, when the sun is low in the sky, are the safest times. Too much sun can cause skin cancer.

It is common that people who live in the northern climes do not obtain enough vitamin D. That happened to me and I believe it was what caused peripheral neuropathy in both of my feet. Blood analyses showed my vitamin D level to be very low. Most every day I now take 400 units of vitamin D in addition to the 50 units in the multivitamin.

T is for Temperance. Totally abstain from everything that is harmful: tobacco in all forms, alcohol, caffeine, and unnecessary drugs. Eat nutritious foods in moderation at regular meal times. Avoid snacking.

A is for Air. Enjoy time out in the fresh air each day. If you smoke, make up your mind to quit. The evidence is in. Smoking increases your risk of heart disease, stroke, lung cancer, and bronchitis. Adventist churches have stop-smoking programs to help you quit.

Sleep with your window open. If it is really cold out, crack it open a little. A study was conducted on soldiers living in two army barracks. One was old and drafty; the other was new and air tight. The study showed that the soldiers in the drafty barracks had fewer colds and were healthier than those in the new barracks.

If you have a choice, live in the country. When I was conducting the acid rain research, I learned that city air is much more polluted with an array of contaminants than country air. When we drove from the camp into New York City, I can remember hitting a distinct wall of city air as we neared the city.

R is for Rest. Get a good night's sleep. Aim for seven to nine hours of sleep each night. Without enough sleep, we can not function properly. Go to bed at a reasonable time and you will find yourself rested and refreshed and ready to meet the challenges of a new day. You will sleep better by eating a light meal or no meal close to bedtime. Your stomach needs rest too.

Besides helping us feel rested and better emotionally and physically, sleep helps fight off infection, prevents diabetes, and reduces the risk of heart disease, obesity, and high blood pressure. Sleep is especially important for people with chronic disabilities and disorders such as arthritis, kidney disease, pain, human immunodeficiency virus (HIV), epilepsy, Parkinson's disease, and depression.

Besides a daily rest, we need a weekly rest. God commanded us to work six days a week and to rest on the seventh. Not only do we rest from our normal work routine, but we rest in the knowledge that we do not have to work for our salvation. Jesus has already done the work for us and gives us salvation as a gift. Knowing this, we can truly enjoy a Sabbath day's rest.

T is for Trust in God. In trying to make changes in our lifestyle, we can sometimes become discouraged. It's encouraging to know that we don't have to do it alone. God is our Helper. He not only helps us, but He fills that void inside of us and gives us peace. It is good to know that our Heavenly Father loves us! "And the peace of God, which surpasses all understanding, will guard your hearts and minds through Christ Jesus" (Philippians 4:7).

I believe I am healthier now for starting on these eight preventative health principles 35 years ago. If there are areas in your life where there is room for improvement, I encourage you to set some goals and start working on these principles. You do not have to do them all at once. Set goals that are reasonable. Start on the easiest one and gradually work toward the harder ones. Claim the promise: "I can do all things through Christ who strengthens me" (Phillipians 4:13). You and God are a winning team!

1. http://www.newstart.com

Chapter 18
Back to Washington

"I am the resurrection and the life. He who believes in Me, though he may die, he shall live." - John 11:25

Linda and I missed the Evergreen State and after one and one-half years in Pennsylvania, we decided to move back to Washington. However, I wanted to complete the project I was working on, so we stayed another one and one-half years. As it turned out, I became the only one left of our three-person team. Jerry went back to his home state of Arizona and Terry, the project leader, was promoted to a position in Washington DC.

We changed the scope of the project to simply comparing the ecology of a stained water stream to that of a clear water stream without the addition of limestone. I gave advance notice to the director that I would be leaving when I finished writing the report. He doubted that I would follow through and leave because I already had too much time in with the Service. When the report was almost finished, I gave notice in writing.

A month later we rented a moving van, loaded up all our belongings, and headed back to Washington. I drove the truck with my mother and Heather, and Linda drove the car with Dawn and Jake. We were doing pretty well staying together until Chicago. The traffic there was very heavy, and we became separated, each going a different way. This was before cell phones and I thought: *it is going to be a while before I see Linda again.* But after leaving Chicago and the worst of the traffic, I spotted a rest area up ahead and pulled in. To my joy and amazement, there were Linda, Dawn, and Jake. We were together again and stayed that way for the rest of our trip.

While in Pennsylvania, we were renting our house in Washington with the plan of retiring there someday. So we had a house to live in when we arrived in Washington. What we did not have were jobs, but in about three weeks Linda found employment in her field of occupational therapy. It took me five years to find employment in my field. During that time, I home-schooled Dawn and Heather and did some handyman jobs on the island. In 1992, Jefferson County hired me to monitor water quality in Jefferson County's streams. Two years later, the work shifted to the Jefferson County Conservation District and I shifted with the work. Twenty-six years later, I am still enjoying working for the Conservation District as I monitor water quality and fish in the streams of Jefferson County.

The Death of My Mother

By this time my mother was getting up in years and she came to live next door to us. Since she was no longer going to the camp, we had to decide what to do with it. At one time in my life the camp was the closest thing to Heaven on earth and I never would have considered selling it, but now I knew I was on track for the real Heaven and New Earth. Even still, it was not easy to do, but we made the decision to sell it. A few years later, my mother's health declined and someone had to stay with her. As it turned out, it was me who was staying with her when she died peacefully in her sleep.

Where did my mother go when she died? In my early years in Catholic schools, I was taught that, when a person died, he/she went to one of three places: Heaven, Hell, or Purgatory. Going to Heaven was to be with God and the angels somewhere "up" beyond the sky. I imagined Hell to be somewhere "down" in the earth where everything is fiery and molten. When I prayed the Apostles' Creed and said the words "He [Jesus] descended into Hell and on the third day He rose again from the dead," I wondered: *why did Jesus go to Hell and what was He doing there for those three days.* The explanation is very simple. The Greek word "Hades," usually translated "Hell," can also be translated "grave" as it is in 1 Corinthians 15:55 (KJV): "O death, where is thy sting? O grave, where is thy victory?" Jesus was in the grave for those three days.

I was taught that Purgatory was like Hell, a burning place of fire. The only difference was that in Purgatory, after a certain length of time based on one's sins, the person would enter Heaven. The length of time in Purgatory could be shortened by friends and loved ones earning "indulgences" for the deceased person. Different prayers were worth various amounts of time off one's stay in Purgatory. Having a Mass said for the person was worth a lot of time off. I remember going to the Rectory with an offering to have a Mass said for a deceased person and getting a Mass card to give to the person's relative.

It was the practice of selling indulgences that stirred Martin Luther, a Catholic priest, into speaking out against this unbiblical tradition. In Luther's day, one could even buy indulgences for future sins! The money gained from this practice financed the building of the magnificent and expensive cathedrals. In 1517, Luther nailed his "ninety-five theses" of protest to the door of the Wittenberg church and the Protestant Reformation began.

As a young man in my twenties, I was bothered by the unfairness of indulgences. A person with many relatives and friends would have his time in Purgatory shortened by indulgences, but a person without any friends or relatives would have to suffer the entire time. Nowhere in the Bible is such a system mentioned.

What the Bible Says About Death

The Bible tells us that death is not the end, that everyone who dies will be resurrected, but not all at the same time. Revelation 20 tells us that there will be two resurrections with a thousand years in between. Those that have accepted Jesus as their Lord and Savior will be in the first resurrection. They will be raised with glorified, immortal bodies that will never get sick, hurt, or wear out.

There will be people in Heaven that have not had the opportunity to have heard of Jesus, but He will still be their Savior. They have lived their lives following the promptings of the Holy Spirit, and after they are resurrected, they will meet Jesus and thank Him for being the "Lamb slain from the foundation of the world" (Revelation 13:8).

What happens to a person in the interval between his death and resurrection? The Bible says he goes to sleep. Over and over again, when a king died, the Bible says, "He slept with his fathers" (1 and 2 Kings). Jesus referred to death as a sleep. In Matthew 9:24, when Jesus went to raise a ruler's young daughter from the dead, He said, "Make room, for the girl is not dead, but sleeping."

Likewise, Jesus referred to the death of Lazarus as a sleep: "'Our friend Lazarus sleeps, but I go that I may wake him up.' Then His disciples said, 'Lord, if he sleeps he will get well.' However, Jesus spoke of his death, but they thought that He was speaking about taking rest in sleep. Then Jesus said to them plainly, 'Lazarus is dead'" (John 11:11–14). Lazarus had been dead for four days (John 11:39). Was Lazarus in Heaven during those four days? We do not hear Lazarus saying anything about what it was like in Heaven. If Lazarus was in Heaven, I would think he would have plenty to say including, "Why did you bring me back here?"

Jesus referred to death as a sleep for a good reason. When a person dies, it is like being in a dreamless sleep. A dead person has no consciousness. Ecclesiastes 9:5 says: "For the living know that they will die; but the dead know nothing." Psalm 146:4 says: "His spirit departs, he returns to his earth; in that very day his plans (thoughts, KJV) perish." Psalm 115:17 (NIV) says: "It is not the dead who praise the LORD, those who go down to the place of silence."

If people went immediately to Heaven when they died, we would expect King David to be there because he was a man after God's own heart (Acts 13:22). But Peter, speaking to the crowd at Pentecost, declared that David is dead and buried and did not ascend to heaven (Acts 2:29, 34).

Even Jesus, during the three days He lay in the tomb, had not been to Heaven to see His Father. When Mary Magdalene attempted to hold Jesus on resurrection morning, Jesus said to her, "Do not cling to Me, for I have not yet ascended to My Father" (John 20:17).

Now you may be thinking, as I once did, of a Bible verse that says just the opposite. Did not Jesus promise one of the thieves on the cross that he would be with Him in Paradise that very day? Here is the verse: "And Jesus said to him [the thief], 'Assuredly, I say to you, today you will be with Me in Paradise'" (Luke 23:43). Thirty-six years ago, Pastor Skip explained this apparent contradiction to me. As in Hebrew, Greek has no punctuation. It was added by the translators. If the comma is placed after the word "today," there is no contradiction with what Jesus told Mary. "And Jesus said to him [the thief], 'Assuredly, I say to you today, you will be with Me in Paradise'" When Jesus returns and the thief who believed in Him comes out of the grave, Jesus will escort him along with all the other raised saints to Paradise.

Are there any people in Heaven now? Yes there are. Enoch was the first person that went to Heaven. The Bible says: "Enoch walked with God; and he was not, for God took him" (Genesis 5:24). Elijah and Moses are also there. We know this because they came to speak encouraging words to Jesus when he was transfigured on the mountain (Matthew 17:1–3). Elijah was taken to Heaven without seeing death (2 Kings 2:11) and represents the "saved" who will be alive when Jesus returns. Moses was resurrected from the grave (Jude 9) and represents the "saved" who will be awaked from their "sleep." Finally, there were those who rose from the dead when Jesus "yielded up His spirit" on the cross (Matthew 27:50–53). When one correctly understands that the dead are sleeping and have no consciousness, the resurrection is much better appreciated for the glorious event that it will be!

My mother's death made a great impact on my life. To begin with, I became very angry, but not at God. I became angry at the devil. At this point in my life, I understood the great controversy between Jesus and the devil. I was angry at the devil for bringing death and suffering to our world and I vowed to fight against the devil and to fight against death with all my energy. How does one fight the devil and death? The answer is by carrying out the great commission that Jesus gave to all His disciples—taking the gospel to every kindred, tongue, and people (Matthew 28:16–20).

From the day of my baptism, I became active in the church, but now my activity increased. Much of my non-working, non-sleeping hours are spent doing whatever I can to "fight the good fight." At this very moment I am writing this book! As I write, I am praying for the Holy Spirit to give me the words that will convince you that Jesus has paid the death penalty for your sins and that you can live with Him forever on the New Earth by accepting Him as your Lord and Savior.

Chapter 19

The Truth about Hell

The way of life winds upward for the wise,
That he may turn away from hell below. - Proverbs 15:24

What happens to the people who are not raised and taken to Heaven when Jesus returns? They simply keep on sleeping for another thousand years. They are completely unaware of the passage of time.

How about the "unsaved" people who are alive when Jesus returns? What happens to them? Revelation 6:15–17 says: "And the kings of the earth, the great men, the rich men, the commanders, the mighty men, every slave and every free man, hid themselves in the caves and in the rocks of the mountains, and said to the mountains and rocks, 'Fall on us and hide us from the face of Him who sits on the throne and from the wrath of the Lamb! For the great day of His wrath has come, and who is able to stand?'" They are consumed by the "brightness of His coming" (2 Thessalonians 2:8) for He is a "consuming fire" (Deuteronomy 4:24; Hebrews 12:29). At the coming of Jesus, they go to sleep and join those still in the grave for one thousand more years of sleep.

During this thousand-year period often referred to as the millennium, Satan and the other evil angels are out of the deceiving business because there are no people left alive to deceive. Figuratively speaking, Satan is "bound" for a thousand years (Revelation 20:2). He will "deceive the nations no more till the thousand years [are] finished" (Revelation 20:3). The rest of verse three says: "But after these things he must be released for a little while." He is released when the second resurrection occurs (Revelation 20:5) because now he has people to deceive again

(Revelation 20:7–8). This he wastes no time in doing. He deceives them into believing they can capture New Jerusalem, which has come down from heaven (Revelation 20:9; 21:2). At this point, fire comes down from God out of Heaven and devours them (Revelation 20:9). This is the lake of fire known as hell and is the second death (Revelation 20:14).

One of the devil's biggest lies, aimed directly at the character of God, is that God burns people forever as I was taught in childhood. One can see that hell does not burn forever by letting the Bible answer these two questions: "Where is hell and when is hell?" Revelation 20 answers both of these questions. The lake of fire occurs on the surface of the earth shortly after the second resurrection.

Those raised in the second resurrection are "devoured" by the fire as they attempt to capture the Holy City, New Jerusalem (Revelation 20:9). They are brought to ashes and cease to exist. Malachi 4:1–3 says: "'For behold, the day is coming, burning like an oven, and all the proud, yes, all who do wickedly will be stubble. And the day which is coming shall *burn them up*' says the LORD of hosts, 'that will leave them neither root nor branch. But to you who fear My name the Sun of Righteousness shall arise with healing in His wings; and you shall go out and grow fat like stall-fed calves. You shall trample the wicked, for they shall be *ashes* under the soles of your feet on the day that I do this,' says the LORD of hosts." Obadiah 16 says: "And they *shall be as though they had never been.*" (All preceding emphasis is mine.)

The devil suffers the same fate in the fire. Ezekiel 28:18, 19 says: "You defiled your sanctuaries by the multitude of your iniquities, by the iniquity of your trading; therefore I brought fire from your midst; it *devoured* you, and I turned you to *ashes* upon the earth in the sight of all who saw you. All who knew you among the peoples are astonished at you; you have become a horror, and *shall be no more forever.*" John 3:16 says: "For God so loved the world that He gave His only begotten Son, that whoever believes in Him should *not perish* but have everlasting life." One can deduce that those who do not believe in Jesus *will perish* and will *not* have everlasting life. (All preceding emphasis is mine.)

God is a God of love! (1 John 4:8, 16). His having to destroy the people He created is referred to as a "strange act" (Isaiah 28:21). It is in mercy that God allows people who are not going to change and who would not enjoy living in God's kingdom to go to sleep and not wake up.

The lake of fire that consumes people is the fire that Peter wrote about that melts every thing down to its basic elements (2 Peter 3:10–12). It is after this, when all of the saints are watching from New Jerusalem, that Jesus makes everything new, never to suffer from the blight of sin again! (Nahum 1:9). Revelation 21:3 says that God will dwell with us on the New Earth. It does not make sense for God and His people to be living on the earth at the same time the "unsaved" are burning in a lake of fire. After the fire turns everything to ashes the fire goes out and God creates everything new! Then the words spoken by Jesus on the mountain come true: "Blessed are the meek, for they shall inherit the earth" (Matthew 5:5).

The verse that makes it appear that the fire burns forever is Revelation 14:11: "And the smoke of their torment ascends forever and ever." The word "forever" in the Bible does not always mean "without end." The Bible sometimes uses the word "forever" in association with things coming to an end. For instance, in Exodus 21:6, a servant is said to serve his master "forever," but this obviously means for the servant's lifetime. Similarly, in 1 Samuel 1:22, 28 when Samuel's mother offered Samuel to serve in God's house "forever," she meant for "as long as he lives." Sodom and Gomorrah were said to suffer the vengeance of "eternal fire," but we know that the fire has gone out (Jude 9).

Part of the problem for thinking that God burns people forever has to do with another of Satan's deceptions that crept into the church centuries ago through Greek philosophers. It is the belief that humans are born immortal. If humans never die and are not saved, they have to be somewhere. This mistaken belief has led to the misconception of an eternal hell fire. However, the Bible is very clear that we are not naturally immortal. Only the saved are given immortality at the time of the first resurrection when Jesus returns. The apostle Paul wrote: "Behold, I tell you a mystery: We shall not all sleep, but we shall all be changed—in a moment, in the twinkling of an eye, at the last trumpet. For the trumpet will sound, and the dead will be raised incorruptible, and we shall be changed. For this corruptible must put on incorruption, and this *mortal* must put on immortality" (1 Corinthians 15:51–53). Those raised in the second resurrection do not put on immortality. Only God is naturally immortal as Paul wrote: "King of kings and Lord of lords, *who alone has immortality"* (1 Timothy 6:15, 16). (All preceding emphasis is mine.)

As one can see, death, resurrection, hell, and immortality are interrelated; misunderstanding one leads to misunderstanding another. To start unraveling falsehoods brought into the Christian church centuries ago, start with something very basic. The Bible says God is love (1 John 4:8, 16). Proof of this love is in the other-centered love demonstrated by God in giving His Son to the human race. To save us from experiencing the second death, Jesus came to earth as a human being to suffer and die and taste the second death Himself (Hebrews 2:9). Actions do speak louder than words. As we consider the cross of Calvary, there should be no doubt about God's love for us!

If a parent needs to discipline a child to correct a bad behavior, what parent would spank the child without stopping? Neither would a loving God keep on burning people without stopping. The second death, spoken of in Revelation 20, is a permanent sleep. There is no resurrection from the second death. As mentioned previously, the unsaved angels and humans *will be no more forever* (Ezekiel 28:18, 19; Malachi 4:1; Obadiah 16).

Think about this. There will be some people that are saved that have family members who are not saved. Could the saved be happy knowing that their husband or wife or child is continually suffering? The concept of a continually burning hell comes straight from Satan, a "liar and the father of lies" (John 8:44).

Chapter 20

Spiritualism, Deception, and Other Snares of Satan

*And when they say to you, "Seek those who are mediums and wizards,
who whisper and mutter," should not a people seek their God? Should they
seek the dead on behalf of the living?* - Isaiah 8:19

Having a correct understanding of what happens to people when they die is important. The Bible tells us that angels have the ability to look like humans. The angels that destroyed Sodom and Gomorrah appeared to Lot as men (Genesis 19:15). Mary Magdalene spoke with two angels who looked like men at Jesus' tomb (John 20:12, 13). In both of these examples, the angels that appeared as men were good angels, but evil angels can and do appear as humans. In *The Great Controversy* (page 552),[1] Ellen White has pointed out the danger of believing that the dead are not really dead:

> He [Satan] has power to bring before men the appearance of their departed friends. The counterfeit is perfect; the familiar look, the words, the tone, are reproduced with marvelous distinctness. Many are comforted with the assurance that their loved ones are enjoying the bliss of Heaven, and without suspicion of danger, they give ear "to seducing spirits, and doctrines of devils."
>
> When they have been led to believe that the dead actually return to communicate with them, Satan causes those to appear

who went into the grave unprepared. They claim to be happy in Heaven and even to occupy exalted positions there, and thus the error is widely taught that no difference is made between the righteous and the wicked. The pretended visitants from the world of spirits sometimes utter cautions and warnings which prove to be correct. Then, as confidence is gained, they present doctrines that directly undermine faith in the Scriptures. With an appearance of deep interest in the well-being of their friends on earth, they insinuate the most dangerous errors. The fact that they state some truths, and are able at times to foretell future events, gives to their statements an appearance of reliability; and their false teachings are accepted by the multitudes as readily, and believed as implicitly, as if they were the most sacred truths of the Bible.

Satan Impersonates Christ

The most powerful of all impersonations that is sure to deceive millions of unknowing people is yet to come. "For Satan himself transforms himself into an angel of light" (2 Corinthians 11:14). In *The Great Controversy* (page 624),[1] Ellen White describes what will be Satan's most masterful deception:

> As the crowning act in the great drama of deception, Satan himself will personate Christ. The church has long professed to look to the Saviour's advent as the consummation of her hopes. Now the great deceiver will make it appear that Christ has come. In different parts of the earth, Satan will manifest himself among men as a majestic being of dazzling brightness, resembling the description of the Son of God given by John in the Revelation (Revelation 1:13–15). The glory that surrounds him is unsurpassed by anything that mortal eyes have yet beheld. The shout of triumph rings out upon the air: "Christ has come! Christ has come!" The people prostrate themselves in adoration before him, while he lifts up his hands and pronounces a blessing upon them, as Christ blessed His

disciples when He was upon the earth. His voice is soft and subdued, yet full of melody. In gentle, compassionate tones he presents some of the same gracious, heavenly truths which the Saviour uttered; he heals the diseases of the people, and then, in his assumed character of Christ, he claims to have changed the Sabbath to Sunday, and commands all to hallow the day which he has blessed. He declares that those who persist in keeping holy the seventh day are blaspheming his name by refusing to listen to his angels sent to them with light and truth. This is the strong, almost overmastering delusion.

Ellen White goes on to say, "The people of God will *not* be misled." God does not give Satan permission to come in the manner that the Bible describes Christ's return. When Christ returns, "every eye will see Him" (Revelation 1:7) and we will meet Him "*in the air*" (1 Thessalonians 4:17; all emphasis mine). Anyone walking on this earth who claims to be Christ is an impostor.

False Healings

Impersonating deceased people and Christ himself is not the only way Satan and his evil angels will attempt to deceive us. A number of years ago I heard Will Baron speak at a church camp meeting. Will, a refrigerator repairman from California, had written a book, *Deceived by the New Age.*[2] In his testimony at camp meeting, Will told how he was made sick until he deposited money to an account tied to Satan's priests. As soon as Will deposited the money, the pain left him. This was done several times until his bank account was depleted. When that happened, he was instructed to use his credit card.

Ellen White wrote about evil angels making people sick and then miraculously healing them:

Men under the influence of evil spirits will work miracles. They will make people sick by casting their spell upon them, and will then remove the spell, leading others to say that those who were sick have been miraculously healed. This Satan has done again and again.

The sick will be healed before us. Miracles will be performed in our sight. Are we prepared for the trial which awaits us when the lying wonders of Satan shall be more fully exhibited? [3]

Satan's Use of Music

Satan, who was created with "timbrels and pipes" (Ezekiel 28:13), uses music to benumb the senses, making it difficult for people to make right decisions. Referring to what took place at a church camp meeting in Indiana in connection to a fanatical "holy flesh" movement, Ellen White wrote:

> The things you have described as taking place in Indiana, the Lord has shown me would take place just before the close of probation. Every uncouth thing will be demonstrated. There will be shouting, with drums, music, and dancing. The senses of rational beings will become so confused that they cannot be trusted to make right decisions.
>
> A bedlam of noise shocks the senses and perverts that which if conducted aright might be a blessing. The powers of satanic agencies blend with the din and noise to have a carnival, and this is termed the Holy Spirit's working. . . . Those things which have been in the past will be in the future. Satan will make music a snare by the way in which it is conducted. [3]

False Religious Leaders

Throughout the ages Satan has enlisted religious leaders to deceive the people. In Jesus' day the people put their trust in the Pharisees and Sadducees. Many thought that Jesus was the Messiah, but because the religious leaders rejected Him, they too rejected Him. Thankfully, after hearing Peter speak on Pentecost Day of the resurrected Jesus, three thousand expressed their faith in Jesus by being baptized (Acts 2:36-41).

From the beginning of the Christian church, Satan has used Christian leaders to introduce false teachings into the church. That is why there was need for the Reformation.

Books and movies, such as the *Left Behind* series, expand the reach of false teachings. It is pleasing to think that you will be whisked away to Heaven before the tribulation occurs. And it is reassuring to believe that if you are not in the group that is whisked away, you will be given a second chance. From my study of the Bible, I do not believe that either one of these teachings is true. For something as important as your eternal salvation, it is foolish to trust it to a minister. I encourage you to prayerfully study God's word for yourself. As God reveals something to you, put it into practice and He will reveal more and more.

Keep false religious leaders in mind when you read about climate change in Chapter 25.

False Science

Satan was the mastermind behind Charles Darwin's book *Origin of Species*. Evolution is now taught as fact in our public schools starting in the earliest grades. Many people have accepted it unquestionably because it is promulgated by the world's leading scientists. But if something is false, even if all the world's most credentialed scientists say it is true, it is still false. Evolution is in direct opposition to the true account of our origin as recorded in the Bible.

It is understandable why some people like the concept of evolution. If we are here by chance, we are not accountable to a Creator God—no worry about a coming judgment.

Pantheism

Pantheism—believing that God is in all things—is another belief system to divert people from the truth. In the words of Ellen White:

> The theory that God is an essence pervading all nature is one of Satan's most subtle devices. It misrepresents God and is a dishonor to His greatness and majesty.
>
> Pantheistic theories are not sustained by the word of God. The light of His truth shows that these theories are soul-destroying agencies. Darkness is their element, sensuality their

sphere. They gratify the natural heart and give license to inclination. Separation from God is the result of accepting them.

Our condition through sin has become preternatural, and the power that restores us must be supernatural, else it has no value. There is but one power that can break the hold of evil from the hearts of men, and that is the power of God in Jesus Christ. Only through the blood of the Crucified One is there cleansing from sin. His grace alone can enable us to resist and subdue the tendencies of our fallen nature. This power the spiritualistic theories concerning God make of no effect. If God is an essence pervading all nature, then He dwells in all men; and in order to attain holiness, man has only to develop the power that is within him.

These theories, followed to their logical conclusion, sweep away the whole Christian economy. They do away with the necessity for the atonement and make man his own savior.[4]

Deception—Satan's Most Powerful Weapon

Deception is Satan's most powerful weapon. It brought down Adam and Eve and turned paradise on earth into a decaying planet. "You will not surely die," the serpent (Satan) said to Eve (Genesis 3:4). If Eve had not fallen for the lie, how different things would be on planet earth. There would be no contaminants in our food, no sickness, no doctors, no hospitals, no policemen, no prisons, and no death.

That lie—"You will not surely die"—was the beginning of Satan's deceptive artistry on earth, but it was not his first lie. His first lie was told in Heaven! From Revelation 12:7–9, we read: "And *war* broke out in heaven: Michael and his angels fought with the dragon; and the dragon and his angels fought, but they did not prevail, nor was a place found for them in heaven any longer. So the great dragon was cast out, that serpent of old, called the Devil and Satan, *who deceives the whole world*; he was cast to the earth, and his angels were cast out with him" (emphasis mine).

The Greek word *war* is "polemos." It can also be translated dispute, quarrel, or strife. It is similar to our words *policy* and *politics*. The war in Heaven between Michael (Jesus) and His angels and Satan and his angels was not conducted with swords or guns, but with words. Satan, insinuating that God was not fair, instigated strife among the angels.

Through deception, Satan gained the allegiance of one-third of all the angels in Heaven and they were cast out with him to this earth. We gain insight that it was Satan's lies that deceived the angels when we read, "His *tail* drew a third of the *stars* of heaven and threw them to the earth" (Revelation 12:4). *Stars* represent angels (Revelation 1:20). *Tail* represents "lies" (Isaiah 9:15). Have you ever heard anyone tell a "tall tail"? Satan was the originator of lies. That is why Jesus called him the "father of it [lies]" (John 8:44).

The Bible, a Safeguard

Here is where an understanding of the Bible is of the utmost importance and why you should *make* time to prayerfully study it like your eternal life depends on it. Heed God's warning made through His last-day prophet in *The Great Controversy* (pages: 625–626):[1]

Only those who have been diligent students of the Scriptures and who have received the love of the truth will be shielded from the powerful delusion that takes the world captive. By the Bible testimony these will detect the deceiver in his disguise. To all the testing time will come. By the sifting of temptation the genuine Christian will be revealed. Are the people of God now so firmly established upon His word that they would not yield to the evidence of their senses? Would they, in such a crisis, cling to the Bible and the Bible only? Satan will, if possible, prevent them from obtaining a preparation to stand in that day. He will so arrange affairs as to hedge up their way, entangle them with earthly treasures, cause them to carry a heavy, wearisome burden, that their hearts may be overcharged with the cares of this life and the day of trial may come upon them as a thief.

1. White, E. G. 1911. *The Great Controversy.* Review and Herald Publishing Association, Mountain View, California.

2. Baron, Will. 1991. *Deceived by the New Age.* Pacific Press Publishing Association, Nampa, Idaho.

3. Widicker, B. (editor). 1992. *Last Day Events: Facing Earth's Final Crisis.* Compiled from the writings of Ellen G. White, Pacific Press Publishing Association, Boise, Idaho, 159, 166.

4. White, E. 1948. *Testimonies for the Church*, Volume 8, Pacific Press Publishing Association, Boise, Idaho, 291.

Chapter 21

Providential Encounters

And we know that all things work together for good to them that love God, to them who are the called according to his purpose. - Romans 8:28

KROH—Radio of Hope

In 2007, I developed peripheral neuropathy in both legs. It started out very painful and I was having a hard time sleeping. Late one night while lying on the sofa and watching programs on 3ABN (Three Angels Broadcasting Network),[1] I heard that the Federal Communications Commission (FCC) was accepting applications for new radio stations.

Every church should be taking advantage of this, I thought. Then it occurred to me, *Who is going to start a radio station in Port Townsend?*

There was only a one-week period that the FCC was accepting applications and it was only two months away. I felt impressed to do something, but kept thinking, *Is God really speaking to me?* The only thing I knew about radio was how to turn one on and adjust the dial.

I did a lot of serious praying about it and asked God, "Do You really want me to do something?"

The Great Commission of spreading the gospel (Matthew 28:16–20) kept coming to my mind. I knew it was God's will to spread the gospel every way that we possibly can, and I started moving forward.

In Search of a Frequency

The first step was to find out if there was a frequency available in the Port Townsend area. My friend Dan Cotton knew a radio engineer at Life Talk Radio and Dan asked him to find out if there was a frequency not being used. After doing some research, the engineer said that it did not look promising, but that a good engineer might possibly be able to squeeze one in. Due to the nearness of the deadline, it took three phone calls before finding an engineer willing to take on the project. After doing his work, the engineer found only one frequency that would work — 91.1. When you need help, what number do you call? 911! What divine providence that such a memorable and significant number was the *only* frequency available!

So far, I had not approached the Port Townsend Church about taking on a radio station. It was now time to find out if the church would commit to building a radio station. The Port Townsend Church is a small church and I was apprehensive about what the church board would say. At the next board meeting I introduced the idea and the discussion began. I slumped lower and lower in my chair as reason after reason was given as to why it could not be done. But then, unexpectedly, the person who had been the most negative took a 180-degree turn and began speaking in favor of it! A motion to apply for a radio station was made and seconded and when the votes were counted, the motion passed!

Looking for a Tower Site

Now the work began. The engineer had used a hypothetical tower site in determining if a frequency was available, but the FCC required an actual location. Ed Sherman, a ham radio friend, recommended that I call another ham. Ed's friend told me that Blyn Mountain, ten miles from Port Townsend, was the best place to have a tower. There was already an "antenna farm" on top of this 2,000-foot high mountain that was used by the Navy, Coast Guard, State Patrol, Jefferson County, and Verizon.

The next clear day, Ed and I drove up the mountain on a winding road past two iron gates that are normally closed and locked. However, on this day both gates were open and we made it to the top. Surrounded by towers, it seemed like another world up there. A technician working on equipment pointed us to a tower belonging to a company that leased antenna space.

I contacted the company and secured a letter granting us space for an antenna at the thirty-foot level. Although this letter satisfied the FCC application, it turned out that our directional antenna required ten feet of clearance all around it and there was no place on the tower that met this requirement.

The only alternative was to lease a plot of land from the Department of Natural Resources and build our own tower. But where would we build it? The small area on the mountain top was already crowded with towers. We attempted to place our tower near Jefferson County's tower, but a consultant who was planning to add 20 feet to the county's tower objected.

Then I discovered a plateau a little lower in elevation off to one side of the antenna farm. But exactly where on the plateau would it be located without blocking signals from the numerous dishes on all the towers? After carefully examining the direction that each dish was pointing, I found a location that did not appear to be blocking any of their signals. However, there was one more potential problem. The 20-foot extension on Jefferson County's tower had not been installed yet and this extension was to have four dishes mounted on it. It was hard enough finding a location not in the way of the dishes I could see, but now I had to contend with dishes that were not installed yet!

Before telling how this was accomplished, I need to back up about 20 years. When I returned to Washington, I took some training in being a colporteur or literature evangelist. I persuaded my friend Norm Houck into accompanying me and we drove around the countryside selling and giving away Christian paperback books. One day we drove up a particularly steep driveway in which the center of the road had been washed out. The farther we went, the worse the road became and I wondered if we should back up. After going more than a mile we came to a house on top of the hill. The house belonged to Bud Brewer, a surveyor and we left a few books with him. Over the years I ran into Bud now and then. One of those encounters occurred when we were starting work on the radio station. I was telling Bud about the station when he commented that I might be in need of a surveyor, and if I did, to let him know.

The time had now come so I visited Bud and told him about our situation on the mountain. Bud knew just what to do. He surveyed the location of Jefferson County's tower and obtained the azimuths of the signal paths of the four uninstalled dishes. With this information Bud calculated the coordinates of a location that would not interfere with Jefferson County's signals. I submitted the tower coordinates to the FCC. After several months of waiting, the FCC issued a construction permit.

Finding Workers

The questions now were, "Who is going to draw up plans? And who is going to do the building?"

Then I thought about our annual church camp meeting in Auburn, Washington where five thousand people would gather together in Rainier Auditorium. I thought about calling the Washington Conference and asking for some time to speak, but my timidity prevailed and I did not.

In the middle of the ten-day Camp Meeting, my path crossed with John Freedman, the conference president. I told him what was on my heart.

He said, "You could have the prayer for the offering tomorrow night and could say a few words about the radio station."

When the time came, there was not enough room for me on the platform and I was invited back the following night. The following night the same thing happened, but this time I was offered a full five minutes to speak during Sabbath School on the last day of camp meeting.

What to Say?

It has been my custom each year at camp meeting to take a walk down to the Green River, sit on a log, and pray. This time I had a lot to pray about. What was I going to say in five minutes? I brought a note pad with me and made a lot of notes.

To say I was nervous would be a great understatement. I am not a public speaker. In four years of high school, only once did I do any public speaking. It was a debate in my economics class. I had my entire speech written out and was reading it word for word. Knowing that a speaker should look at the audience once in a while, I looked up. When I looked back at my script, I could not find my place! It seemed like an hour went by before I found it and I did not look up again.

In college, I was required to take public speaking, and every time I spoke, I was scared to death. Once I stood up to speak and could not remember my topic!

The Miracle

Now here is the miracle. Sabbath morning came and I stood up to speak in front of a packed auditorium. As soon as I opened my mouth, the Holy Spirit took control and words came out. I knew it was not really me speaking.

At the break between Sabbath School and worship service, people came up to me saying they would help. Grady Stevens, a retired architect from the Bellevue church, was the first to offer his help. Grady made several trips to the tower site and drew up the plans for the equipment shed. He also came to the Jefferson County Planning Department meetings and shepherded the plans through the permitting process. Gail Kiele of the Bremerton Church volunteered her husband Scott, an electrician and owner of George's Electric in Port Orchard. Scott did the wiring at the tower site and the studio.

Closer to home, members of the Port Townsend, Sequim, Poulsbo, and Port Angeles churches came out in force to build the tower and equipment shed. Two ladies, both named Linda, drove a pickup truck pulling a trailer to Portland and brought back the entire disassembled 80-foot tower. Wayne Christensen, a retired civil engineer, oversaw the construction. We assembled the tower in Wayne's backyard, moved it to the site in 20-foot sections, and reassembled it there. Wayne brought his heavy equipment up to the site and dug the foundations for the tower, equipment shed, and propane tank.

Wayne also dug a 400-foot trench for the power cable. The trench was to go through an area surrounded by towers, all of which were fed by underground power cables. We had two different cable locators mark the paths of these cables. Wayne operated his backhoe very slowly through this area. When he approached a painted mark, indicating a power cable, he stopped and we very carefully hand-dug around the cable. Thankfully, the only cables the backhoe cut through were old, inactive cables.

Our 80-foot tower was self-standing, meaning that it required no guy wires. Its foundation was an eleven by eleven by five-foot block of concrete containing an enormous amount of one-inch rebar going in every direction. It took three cement trucks to pour the tower, equipment shed, and propane tank foundations.

I looked in the yellow pages of the phone book for a crane company to place the tower on its foundation. I found one with a name I liked—Affordable Crane. When the owner found out it was for a Christian radio station, he said, "There will be no charge for that."

Most of the construction took place during winter in snow and wind. That 2000 feet of elevation made a chilly difference; it seemed like it went from summer to winter from the bottom to the top of the mountain. On those cold days, everyone looked forward to the hot soup that Linda provided. Frequently, it was lentil soup and I received a lot of good-hearted kidding. "What? Lentils again?"

Those days on the mountain were some of the best days of my life and will be etched in my memory forever. There is something about men and women working together to advance God's cause that satisfies like nothing else can. Most of the people I had never met before, but now I count as true friends.

When God's People Work Together

Last week (March 20, 2019), our Wednesday night prayer group began studying the book of Acts. What an inspiring book to show what God can do through His people when they are filled with the Holy Spirit. Based on the book of Acts, Ellen White wrote *The Acts of the Apostles.*[2] The following is from the first chapter:

> The church is God's appointed agency for the salvation of men. It was organized for service, and its mission is to carry the gospel to the world. From the beginning it has been God's plan

that through His church shall be reflected to the world His fullness and His sufficiency. The members of the church, those whom He has called out of darkness into His marvelous light, are to show forth His glory. The church is the repository of the riches of the grace of Christ; and through the church will eventually be made manifest, even to "the principalities and powers in heavenly places," the final and full display of the love of God. Ephesians 3:10.

Enfeebled and defective as it may appear, the church is the one object upon which God bestows in a special sense His supreme regard. It is the theater of His grace, in which He delights to reveal His power to transform hearts.

The members are to find their happiness in the happiness of those whom they help and bless.

Wonderful is the work which the Lord designs to accomplish through His church, that His name may be glorified.

The apostle Paul compared the church to a human body (1 Corinthians 12:12–31). The body is composed of different parts, all of which are necessary for the body to function at optimum capacity. The church is composed of people with different personalities and different skills. It functions at its best when all are present and are using their skills for the good of the whole. The building of KROH is a good example of what can be accomplished when God's people work together.

The devil does not like it when God's people are working together and will use anything to cause discord and division among church members. It makes no difference to the devil whether it is a disagreement over the interpretation of a Bible text or the color of the carpet. If it causes division and results in people leaving the church, Satan has succeeded.

He has tried it with me, but thankfully, I was aware of his tactic and did not fall for it. How about you? Has he managed to separate you from the apple of God's eye, enfeebled though His church may be? If he has, it's time to come home and show the devil who you take your orders from. Heed the words of God's end-time prophet:

> In our separation from one another we are separated from Christ. We want to press together. Oh, how many times, when I have seemed to be in the presence of God and holy angels, I have heard the angel voice saying, "Press together, press together, press together. Do not let Satan cast his hellish shadow between brethren. Press together; in unity there is strength."[3]

Finding a Location for the Studio

We decided that the Better Living Center was the perfect place for the studio. It is owned by the church so there would be no rent, and it had line-of-sight to the tower for easy transmission of the broadcast signal.

Then I received a phone call from a planner in the Port Townsend Planning Department. He had seen a newspaper article about the radio station and our intention to have the studio at the Better Living Center.

He told me, "You cannot have a radio studio at the Better Living Center because it is in a residential zone."

I made an appointment to see the planner. A week later Dan Cotton and I were in his office. I do not recall all that we said, but we asked him to reconsider. He pointed to a stack of applications on his desk and said, "See all these applications? It will be three or four months before I have time to think about your radio station."

However, one week later the planner called and said that because the church already had a community thrift store in the building, they would grandfather in our studio. This was the work of the Holy Spirit. God's people had put forth their effort and the Holy Spirit had worked on the heart of the planner.

Looking for a Station Manager

The radio station was coming together, but who was going to operate it? I put an ad in the Gleaner, the church magazine for the Pacific Northwest. Through a circuitous route, the ad found its way to Joseph

Mann in Wisconsin. Joe had six years of service in the U.S. Army Signal Corps and decades of experience in two-way and commercial radio. As one of the founders of Life Talk Radio, Joe had the experience needed to start a radio station.

In March 2010, while still in Wisconsin, Joe began helping us develop a website as we waited approval from the FCC. In July, he made the move to Washington, bringing much of his own equipment with him, and began setting up the radio station. His wife Pam, daughter Sarah, and boxer-dog Rocky joined him in January 2011. In August 2011, KROH went on the air!

In 2015, we decided to provide Joe with some help and again put an ad in the Gleaner. Again through a circuitous path, Tony Fabian, who was living in Florida, responded. Although Tony had no radio experience, he came with excellent technical and building skills that he put to good use. Interestingly, different people had told Tony that with his deep bass voice, he should be in radio. I love to hear Tony give the weather report, especially when it is for a sunny day!

The Radio Station Today

KROH is heard via the airwaves over a sizable area in Northwest Washington and even reaches into some parts of British Columbia, and it is being listened to in over 200 countries via the Internet. It was built and continues to be operated by donations from listeners. We constantly hear from listeners who have been blessed by the music and life-saving sermons. If you would like a taste of it, you can listen online at RadioOfHope.org.

Romans 8:28 says that "all things work together for good for those that love God and are called according to His purpose." I see the connection between having peripheral neuropathy, being up late at night to hear the FCC announcement, and starting a radio station as a fulfilment of that Bible promise.

The Formula for Success

Over the years and especially during the building of KROH–Radio of Hope, I have learned the formula for success:

Divine Power + Human Effort = Success

I learned this Bible-based formula from Ellen White's writings. In *Patriarchs and Prophets*,[4] she told how Joshua defeated the Amorites. Joshua prayed for the sun to stand still so that the Israelite army would have enough daylight for a complete victory, but Joshua fought as though his success depended upon the Israelite army alone (Joshua 10:1–15).

Another example is found in John 21:1–6. After a fruitless night of fishing, Jesus told the disciples, "Cast the net on the right side of the boat, and you will find some." When they did, they caught a net full of large fish, 153 to be exact. In the *Desire of Ages*,[5] Ellen White comments: "Jesus had a purpose in bidding them cast their net on the right side of the ship. On that side He stood upon the shore. That was the side of faith. If they labored in connection with Him—His divine power combining with their human effort—they could not fail of success."

In building KROH, many people put their minds and muscles into the work, but without God's Holy Spirit influencing people in authority, there would have been no success.

Another Providence in Another Realm

In 2010, another amazing fulfilment of Romans 8:28 occurred at Heather's wedding that started from a short bathroom conversation with Tim Standish, the cousin of my son-in-law Nigel. Tim is a geneticist at the Geoscience Research Institute[6] in Loma Linda, California. Meeting for the first time in the men's room and learning of our common interest, we talked about fish genetics.

Sometime later, I received a call from Lad Allan, producer of Illustra Media's documentary films[7] that demonstrate in beautiful videography that intelligent design is a much better explanation for the beauty and complexity of life than is evolution. Tim was a friend of Lad's and had helped him produce some of his Intelligent Design films. When Lad was looking for a fishery biologist to help with *Living Waters*,[8] Tim referred him to me.

Living Waters combines studies of four magnificent creatures that share an aqueous environment: whales, sea turtles, dolphins, and salmon. Besides original breath-taking footage of these magnificent creatures in the wild, computer animation reveals the intricate design of systems that show:

- how turtles use a built-in compass to navigate over a thousand miles of ocean;
- how dolphins use echolocation to find and capture prey; and
- how salmon are able to detect minute odor molecules to find their stream of origin.

In order to function correctly, each of these systems requires a number of specialized parts. If any one of the parts is missing, the system will not function. In his book *Darwin's Black Box: The Biochemical Challenge to Evolution*,[9] biochemist Michael Behe termed this concept "irreducible complexity." He illustrated this concept with a simple mousetrap having five parts: wooden base, spring, hammer, lever, and catch. All must be present simultaneously for the mousetrap to function.

This concept applies to magnetic-navigation in sea turtles, echolocation in dolphins, and olfaction (smell) in salmon. Unless all the necessary parts are present simultaneously, the system would not function. Until the system is functional so that it provides an advantage for the animal's survival, the genes associated with the necessary parts would not be passed on to the next generation.

Someone said that the reason organisms appear designed is because they *are* designed! Even evolutionary biologist, outspoken atheist, and author Richard Dawkins in his book *The Blind Watchmaker*[10] said, "Yet the living results of natural selection overwhelmingly impress us with the appearance of designs if by a master watchmaker, impress us with the illusion of design and planning."

I believe that it is more than an "illusion"!

What a privilege it was to have a part in *Living Waters*. After Lad and videographer Jerry Harned finished filming sockeye salmon in British Columbia, they came to my house to film me explaining how a salmon returns to its natal stream.

Afterward, I took them to Salmon Creek where summer chum salmon had been spawning. If you watch *Living Waters*, you will see a lone salmon swimming across a riffle. It was the tail end of the spawning season and this salmon was about the last chum salmon still alive.

You can find *Living Waters* and other Illustra Media productions including *Metamorphosis, Origin, Flight, Unlocking the Mystery of Life, The Privileged Planet* and others at the web site www.illustramedia.com. The videography in each of these films is every bit as good as that of National Geographic and the computer animations, depicting the complexity of life, will leave you with no doubt about a Master Designer behind it all.

1. Three Angels Broadcasting Network, https://3abn.org/

2. White, E. G. 1911. *The Acts of the Apostles.* Pacific Press Publishing Association, Mountain View, California, 9, 12, 13.

3. White, E. G. 1958. *Selected Messages*, Book Two, Review and Herald Publishing Association, Washington, DC, 374.

4. White, E. G. 1958. *Patriarchs and Prophets.* Review and Herald Publishing Association, Mountain View, California, 509.

5. White, E. G. 1898. *The Desire of Ages*, Pacific Press Publishing Association, Mountain View, California, 811.

6. https://www.grisda.org/

7. Illustra Media https://illustramedia.com/

8. Living Waters, http://www.livingwatersthefilm.com/

9. Behe, M. J. 1996. *Darwin's Black Box: The Biochemical Challenge to Evolution.* New York: Free Press. ISBN 978-0-684-82754-4. LCCN 96000695. OCLC 34150540.

10. Dawkins, R. 1986. The Blind Watchmaker: Why the Evidence of Evolution Reveals a Universe without Design, Norton & Company, Inc., United Kingdom, 21.

Chapter 22

Restoration

I will give you a new heart and put a new spirit within you; I will take the heart of stone out of your flesh and give you a heart of flesh. - Ezekiel 36:26

Restoration is a key word for Conservation Districts as well as for other natural resource agencies. During the dust bowl era of the 1930s, farming practices used by prairie settlers resulted in severe soil erosion. When a strong west wind blew so much soil into the air that it caused daytime to look like nighttime in Washington DC, Congress formed the Soil Conservation Service.

During that same era, Conservation Districts began forming across the United States. In that era, emphasis was on improving the land for agriculture. To make the land more productive for farming, wetlands were drained, streams were straightened, and trees were removed to the edge of the stream banks. Unfortunately, this work was often done to the detriment of fish and wildlife. Today, much of the work that Conservation Districts do in the Pacific Northwest involves restoring salmon habitat. Districts are now planting trees along streams to provide shade and building fences to exclude livestock. These practices have resulted in cooler water for salmon and less fecal matter with potential pathogens being ingested by shellfish.

On both coasts of the United States, dams have prevented salmon and other migratory fish from reaching upstream spawning grounds. Restoration projects, involving dam removal, are now underway on a number of rivers. Two salmon rivers that I am very familiar with where dams have been removed are the Elwha River in Washington and the Penobscot River in Maine.

The introduction of fish into waterbodies outside their native range has resulted in the need for restoration. In the early days of fishery management, stocking fish in different streams and lakes was a common practice. That is why we have eastern brook trout in streams and lakes in the West; rainbow trout, native to the West, throughout the East; German brown trout from coast to coast; and all five species of Pacific salmon in the Great Lakes. Non-native species have often out-competed native species, reducing or eliminating them. Some states have restoration programs to eliminate or reduce the number of non-natives. For example, methods are being tested to exterminate non-native lake trout in Yellowstone Lake because they compete with native cutthroat trout.[1]

Carp, native to Asia, were transplanted far and wide throughout this country before it was realized that it was not a good idea. Not only are carp detrimental to native fish, they are detrimental to waterfowl. A carp's mouth is angled downward and is ideal for foraging on the bottom. This manner of feeding stirs up bottom sediment and reduces light penetration. Reduced light results in less aquatic vegetation that waterfowl feed on. When I worked at Marrowstone Field Station, we trained young adults in the Youth Conservation Corps to remove carp from McNary National Wildlife Refuge by trapping and seining. In most cases, once a non-native fish becomes established, it is there for good.

The New Earth

On an infinitely larger scale, our entire planet is in need of restoration. The habitat on planet earth began deteriorating from the time that Adam and Eve disobeyed God in the Garden of Eden and thorns and thistles began appearing (Genesis 3:18). Now almost 6,000 years later, our planet is in need of major restoration. As previously mentioned, even our good intentions have resulted in unintended consequences.

The good news is that God has a *major* restoration project planned for planet earth! Jesus has told us that the meek will inherit the earth (Matthew 5:5). The lake of fire will melt this polluted earth down to its basic elements and God will create everything new (2 Peter 3:11, 12; Revelation 20 and 21). The result will be what the Bible calls the "New Earth" (Isaiah 65:17; Revelation 21:1). The Garden of Eden will be restored. There will be no thorns or thistles. There will be no carnivores because there will be no death. The wolf and the lamb will feed together and the lion will eat straw like the ox (Isaiah 65:25). The tree of life, bearing a different kind of fruit every month, will be there (Revelation 22:2). God's throne will be there and we will be able to converse with God our Father and with Jesus our Savior face to face (Revelation 22:4). There will never be a need for another restoration project. God, who knows the end from the beginning, has promised it. Over the eons of time, sin will never ever happen again. (Nahum 1:9). Praise the Lord!

A New Heart

As great as the restoration of the earth will be—and it will be beyond imagination—it is not God's greatest restoration project. His greatest restoration project is the restoration of us! When God created Adam and Eve, He created them "in His own image" (Genesis 1:27). Their character was like God's; they were *other*-centered. When Adam and Eve sinned, their character changed; they became *self*-centered.

Sadly, the entire human race inherited their self-centered character. We come out of the womb that way. It's all about me! Babies cry out their demands. Two-year olds play "no, no, mine!" Adults look out for "number one."

It is God's greatest desire to restore us to His image of *other*-centeredness. There is no greater example of other-centeredness than the Son of God becoming a human being *forever* in order to restore us to His image. As a human, Jesus gave us an example of what an other-centered life looks like. To observe His life, we have only to read about it in Matthew, Mark, Luke, and John. By beholding Jesus, we become like Him (2 Corinthians 3:18).

However, in order to save us, God needed to do more than give us a demonstration on how to live. God's broken law required the death penalty (Romans 6:23). In order to save us, the eternal Son of God paid the death penalty for us. Not only that, but He also lived a perfect life for us.

Not long ago, when I explained to someone how Jesus died in place of us, he said, "That's not fair." He was right. It is not fair. But if our Creator God is willing to accept it as satisfying his law, who are we to argue and why would we want to! It means our salvation!

Besides, there is more to it than simply satisfying the law as the following story demonstrates. A mother discovered that her young son had told a lie. She loved her son and knew she had to correct him. She told him to go out and cut a willow branch and bring it to her. When he returned with it, she held out her arm and told him to hit her with it. He began hitting her lightly, but she insisted that he hit her harder. As her arm turned red and welts began forming, tears streamed down his face. That was the last lie he told. When we realize that we crucify Jesus afresh by our sins, it is a powerful motive for change (Hebrews 6:6).

Besides being self-centered, we are also naturally proud. We all need restoration! That is why Jesus said to Nicodemus, "Unless one is born of water and the Spirit, he cannot enter the kingdom of God" (John 3:5). God's greatest desire is to restore us to His image—to give us a new heart and to put a new spirit within us (Ezekiel 36:26; Hebrews 10:16). He wants to completely transform us into being a "new creation" (2 Corinthians 5:17).

I think this is why God has given us examples of insects that metamorphose from a larva to a completely different-looking adult. A beautiful butterfly looks nothing like the caterpillar it starts out as. Once on an early summer morning as the sun began warming the side of my house, some movement directed my eyes to a cocoon attached to the house. As I watched, a butterfly emerged. What takes place inside the cocoon is amazing. It is not simply a leg or an eye becoming slightly different; everything about the butterfly is completely different from the caterpillar. What occurs is a complete melt down of the caterpillar before the butterfly is formed. Watch *Metamorphosis*[2] and see for yourself!

We cannot change ourselves. It is the work of the Holy Spirit. How do we receive the Holy Spirit? We ask. Read what Jesus said in Luke 11:5–13 and see how much God desires to give us His Holy Spirit.

Keep in mind that it is God who creates in us a new heart, not us. If we look to ourselves to do it, we would say "impossible" and give up. Fortunately, it is almighty God who does the restoring and He is able! If you, like me, think it would take a miracle to change your heart, you are right; but take courage because God is in the miracle business! The Bible says He "is able to do exceedingly abundantly above all that we ask or think, according to the power that works in us" (Ephesians 3:20). That power is the power of grace applied to our hearts (minds) by the Holy Spirit; "with God all things are possible" (Matthew 19:26).

The story of God bringing His people Israel out of slavery in Egypt into the Promised Land symbolizes God bringing us out of slavery to sin into the real Promised Land, the New Earth. God brought His people out by a series of miracles: the crossing of the Red Sea, feeding them manna from Heaven, protecting them from fiery serpents, crossing the Jordan River in flood stage, and causing the walls of Jericho to fall down flat. However, not all the Israelites made it into the Promised Land. Of all the people older than twenty, only Joshua and Caleb entered in. The reason the others did not enter in was because of their *unbelief* (Hebrews 3:19). They feared the giants in their walled cities. They had already forgotten how God had parted the Red Sea and destroyed their enemies.

It is so important to take God at His word and believe that He is able to do what He says *He will do*. This is what God says *He will do*: "This is the covenant I will make with them after that time, says the Lord. *I will put my laws in their hearts,* and *I will write them on their minds*" (Hebrews 10:16). "Let us hold unswervingly to the hope we profess, for *He who promised is faithful*" (Hebrews 10:23, all emphasis is mine). Believing God is so important! Using a Bible concordance, check out the word "believe" and "belief" as used by Jesus. Also, check out its antonym, "unbelief."

God has high expectations of us. Anyone who comes to Him can be saved and restored to His image. He can save to the *uttermost* those who come to Him through Jesus (Hebrews 7:25) and He can create in us new hearts (Ezekiel 36:26). Jesus paid the price for all. "For God so loved the world that He gave His only begotten Son, that *whoever* believes in Him should not perish but have everlasting life" (John 3:16).

When we repent and confess our sins, and believe that Jesus has died for us the death we deserve and has lived the perfect life for us that we have failed to live, at that moment God gives us eternal life. From this point in time, God does not see our sinful life. He sees the perfect life of Jesus. Our salvation is based entirely on accepting what Jesus has accomplished for us. "For by one offering He has perfected forever those who are being sanctified" (Hebrews 10:14). Sanctification—being restored to the image of God— is the work of a lifetime. Day by day, as we behold the beautiful, other-centered life of Jesus, we become more like Him. The transformation of our proud, self-centered heart into a humble, loving, other-centered heart continues for the rest of our lives until our mortal bodies become immortal in the twinkling of an eye at the coming of Jesus (1 Corinthians 15:53). Before that day when our transformation is complete, we can be assured that our "service [for Him] will be accepted, although imperfect"[3] because "Jesus makes up for our unavoidable defiencies."[3] Praise the Lord!

1. Thomas, N. A., C. S. Guy, T. M. Koel, and A. V. Zale. 2019. In-situ evaluation of benthic suffocation methods for suppression of invasive Lake Trout embryos in Yellowstone Lake. *North American Journal of Fisheries Management* 39:104–111.

2. Metamorphosis, https://illustramedia.com/metamorphosis/

3. White, E. G. 1980. *Selected Messages*, Book 3, Review and Herald Publishing Association, Washington, DC, 196.

Chapter 23

Grace Is the Power

having been justified by His grace we should become heirs according to the hope of eternal life. - Titus 3:7

Amazing Grace

Grace has become one of my favorite words along with love, mercy, and forgiveness. It is the antidote for "salvation by works"—trying to earn our way to Heaven. Grace is unearned, unmerited, undeserved favor with God. It is a part of God's unconditional love. God hates sin because it causes our death, but there is nothing we can do to make God stop loving us. The apostle Paul wrote, "Where sin abounded, grace abounded much more" (Romans 5:20). We are saved totally by the life and death of Jesus. As Paul said, "all have sinned and fall short of the glory of God, and all are justified freely by his grace through the redemption that came by Christ Jesus" (Romans 3:23, 24).

Grace is the essence of the gospel. Paul said his ministry was "to testify to the gospel of the grace of God" (Acts 20:24). It bears repeating that our salvation is based entirely on what Jesus has *already accomplished* for us and He gives us salvation as a gift. Paul wrote to the Ephesians: "For by grace you have been saved through faith, and that not of yourselves; it is the *gift* of God, not of works, lest anyone should boast" (Ephesians 2:8, 9; my emphasis).

In her book *The Ministry of Healing*,[1] Ellen White said, "Grace is an attribute of God exercised toward undeserving human beings. We did not seek for it, but it was sent in search of us. God rejoices to bestow His grace upon us, not because we are worthy, but because we are so utterly unworthy. Our only claim to His mercy is our great need."

The Broad Road

Jesus spoke of two roads: a broad road to destruction that many take and a narrow road to eternal life that few take (Matthew 7:13, 14). Ellen White describes those traveling on the broad road:

> The powers of Satan are at work to keep minds diverted from eternal realities. The enemy has arranged matters to suit his own purposes. Worldly business, sports, the fashions of the day—these things occupy the minds of men and women. Amusements and unprofitable reading spoil the judgment. In the broad road that leads to eternal ruin there walks a long procession. The world, filled with violence, reveling, and drunkenness, is converting the church. The law of God, the divine standard of righteousness, is declared to be of no effect.[2]

The Narrow Road

Now let's see what defines the narrow road that leads to eternal life. Jesus said, "I am the *way*, the *truth*, and the *life*. No one comes to the Father except through Me" (John 14:6, emphasis mine). And Luke said, "There is no other name under heaven given among men by which we must be saved" (Acts 4:12). Accepting Jesus as our Savior is paramount to choosing the narrow road that leads to eternal life.

Soon after Jesus spoke about the two roads, He told three short stories. In the first, He told how to recognize a false prophet wearing sheep's clothing (i.e., acting like a Christian by outward appearance). He said you can recognize them by their fruits (Matthew 7:15–20). In the second story, Jesus said, "Not everyone who says to Me, 'Lord, Lord,' shall enter the kingdom of heaven, but he who *does* the will of My Father in heaven" (Matthew 7:21; emphasis mine).

In the third story, Jesus contrasted a wise man from a foolish man by the kind of foundation each built for his house. The wise man built his house on rock and the foolish man built on sand. When the flood came and the winds blew, the house built on sand fell, but the house built on the rock remained standing. Jesus said that the man who built his house on sand was like a man who hears His sayings but does not put them into practice; whereas, the man who built on the rock is like the man who hears His sayings and *does* them (Matthew 7:24–27).

The Ditch of Cheap Grace

These three stories indicate that not all Christians are genuine Christians traveling on the narrow road. The narrow road has two ditches and the devil tries to knock us into one of them. One ditch is believing that once we have accepted Jesus as our Savior, it does not matter what we do afterward. This ditch is sometimes called "once saved, always saved" or "cheap grace." However, being saved by grace and not by keeping the law does not give us free license to sin. Paul writes, "Shall we sin because we are not under law but under grace? Certainly not!" (Romans 6:15).

Sin is destructive and ends in death. God loves us. He created us and knows what is best for us. So that we do not hurt ourselves, He has given us commands on how to live. His commands are simply summed up in the Ten Commandments. Obeying God's commandments is in our own best interest and in the best interest of those around us. We can think of the Ten Commandments as a wall of protection. The Ten Commandments can be summed up in two commandments: loving God with all our heart, soul, strength, and mind and loving our neighbor as our self (Luke 10:27).

Believing in Jesus is essential for our salvation, but we need to understand that this believing is more than just a general acknowledgment that Jesus is real, that He died for the sins of the whole world, and that everything the Bible says about Him is true. Jesus also said, "Most assuredly, I say to you, he who believes in Me, the works that I do he will do also" (John 14:12). We need a personal relationship with Jesus that results in committing our lives to carrying out His will. We are in no way saved by anything we do, but the Bible tells us that what we do with our lives after believing in Jesus and accepting Him as our Savior gives evidence as to the kind of belief or faith we have. What we do does not add anything to what Jesus has accomplished for us.

What we do with our lives results from wanting to please the One who has already saved us and wanting to help others to be saved by accepting the gift of God's grace.

The Ditch of Works

The ditch on the other side of the road is believing that we are partly responsible for our salvation, that our salvation comes from what Jesus did plus what we do. I am sorry to say that not too long after my baptism I fell into this ditch. I have learned that you can identify a person in this ditch by the way he/she is concentrating on doing everything right. The person is highly critical and is not satisfied with himself doing everything right, but wants to make sure everyone else is also doing things right, according to his opinion. In Jesus' day these people were known as Pharisees. I remember Linda saying to me as I arrived home from work one day, "As soon as you come through the door, you start criticizing." I do not know how many years I was in the Pharisee mode, but I am very grateful for a wife who stuck it out during that era of my life when I was not the easiest person to live with.

What is especially bad about being in this ditch is that the person thinks he is just fine. He is blind to his condition. Jesus spoke to people in this condition in His letter to the church of Laodicea. He said, "Because you say, 'I am rich, have become wealthy, and have need of nothing'—and do not know that you are wretched, miserable, poor, blind, and naked" (Revelation 3:17). What opened my eyes to my condition was attending a church camp meeting when the theme that year was "righteousness by faith." I am thankful that we serve a God who is "merciful, gracious, and longsuffering" (Exodus 34:6) and forgiving (1 John 1:9).

The Cart and the Horse

Contrary to the ways of this world in which we work hard to earn a good school grade or promotion, God gives us grace "up-front." As soon as we accept Jesus as our Savior, we have eternal life. There is nothing more to earn! We have it by *believing* that Jesus has paid the death penalty for our sins and lived the perfect life that He credits to our account in the Book of Life (John 5:24; 6:29; 7:38; 11:25, 26). When we really take this home and begin to grasp what this means, a love for God springs up within us. We will be living to please God. The things of this world will no longer have an attraction for us. We will start living to share this good news with others and throw ourselves into God's work. We will be working hard; not to gain what we already have, but to help others to have it. We will not be anxious about anything, but will have the peace that surpasses all understanding.

We are familiar with the expression, "putting the cart ahead of the horse." Doing lots of good deeds in order to merit God's favor is like putting the cart ahead of the horse. Correctly understood, God's grace, represented by the horse, comes first; then comes the cart filled with good works. Good works are the result of God's amazing grace.

The life of Mary of Magdalene is a beautiful example of how grace works. As part of a plan to trap Jesus, Mary had been set up and caught in adultery. The Pharisees brought her to Jesus saying, "Now Moses, in the law, commanded us that such should be stoned. But what do You say?" After Jesus bent down and wrote with His finger on the ground, they were convicted by their conscience and began leaving, beginning with the oldest. When Jesus straightened up and saw no one there but the woman, He said to her, "Woman, where are those accusers of yours? Has no one condemned you?" She said, "No one, Lord." And Jesus said to her, "Neither do I condemn you; go and sin no more" (John 8:1–11). Jesus extended grace to Mary and it changed her life.

It was Mary who sat at Jesus' feet and listened to His every word. At Simon's feast, it was Mary who poured the expensive anointing oil upon Jesus' head, bathed His feet with her tears, and dried them with her hair. It was Mary who stood beside the cross. It was Mary who was first at the empty tomb. And it was Mary who first proclaimed a risen Savior. It was God's grace that changed Mary.

At the 2014 camp meeting in Auburn, I experienced something that never happened to me before and has never happened since. I was walking across the large, grassy area in the center of the campus when the words "Grace is the power" were written across my mind. I heard no voice, but these four words were distinct. I had not been thinking about "grace." In fact, I had not been thinking of anything at all. The words came out of the blue.

Previous to this incident, I was familiar with the word grace. It was not a new word to me, but since that occurrence, I have experienced a deeper appreciation and a deeper understanding of "grace." Grace is the power. It is the power for overcoming selfishness and pride. It is the power for a changed life. Grace up-front. God's love first. It was grace that changed the lives of Mary, Peter, James, John and Paul, and it is grace that is changing my life. My prayer is that you too will experience God's grace and allow it to change your life.

1. White, E. G. 1942. *The Ministry of Healing*, Pacific Press Publishing Association, Mountain View, California, 161.

2. White, E. G. 1948. *Testimonies for the Church*, Pacific Press Publishing Association, Boise, Idaho, 43, 44.

Chapter 24
A Breach in God's Law

You shall be called the Repairer of the Breach. - Isaiah 58:12 (KJV)

The Sabbath, which points us back to creation, and the miraculous manner in which God created everything—by speaking it into existence (Genesis 1)—gives us confidence that He is able to create in us new hearts. Our resting on the Sabbath symbolizes our acceptance of what Jesus has accomplished for us without trying to add anything to it, lest we should boast about it (Ephesians 2:9). It was pride that caused the downfall of Lucifer and God does not want to give us any opportunity to boast!

From the first seven days of creation, the Sabbath was given to us as a weekly reminder that it was God who created the heavens and the earth (Genesis 2:2). God reconfirmed the Sabbath and its connection to creation when He gave the Ten Commandments to Moses and the Israelites at Mount Sinai by speaking and writing them in stone (Exodus 20). The Sabbath commandment is the only one beginning with the word "remember," but it is the commandment that has been forgotten the most. Among most Christians today, Sunday has taken its place. Most Christians will say that Sunday is in recognition of the resurrection, but God did not bless and sanctify the first day of the week and tell us to rest on that day. He did not tell us that He changed the fourth commandment.

Some say that the Sabbath was meant only for the Jews, but God gave the Sabbath to the entire human race during the first week of creation, long before Abraham. The Bible indicates that the Sabbath will still be kept in the future. In speaking of the future "great tribulation," Jesus said to pray that your flight not be on the Sabbath (Matthew 24:20, 21). And Isaiah prophesied that we will be keeping the Sabbath on the New Earth (Isaiah 66:23).

The author of Hebrews said that the sanctuary that God instructed Moses to build was a "copy and shadow" of the sanctuary in Heaven (Hebrews 8:1–5; 9:4). Therefore, we would expect that the Ten Commandments that resided in the ark in the Most Holy Place of the sanctuary built by Moses are a replica of the Ten Commandments residing in the sanctuary in Heaven. This is exactly what Ellen White saw in vision:

> Elder Bates was resting upon Saturday, the seventh day of the week, and he urged it upon our attention as the true Sabbath. I did not feel its importance, and thought that he erred in dwelling upon the fourth commandment more than upon the other nine.
>
> But the Lord gave me a view of the heavenly sanctuary. The temple of God was open in heaven, and I was shown the ark of God covered with the mercy seat. Two angels stood one at either end of the ark, with their wings spread over the mercy seat, and their faces turned toward it. This, my accompanying angel informed me, represented all the heavenly host looking with reverential awe toward the law of God, which had been written by the finger of God.
>
> Jesus raised the cover of the ark, and I beheld the tables of stone on which the ten commandments were written. I was amazed as I saw the fourth commandment in the very center of the ten precepts, with a soft halo of light encircling it. Said the angel, "It is the only one of the ten which defines the living God who created the heavens and the earth and all things that are therein."
>
> When the foundations of the earth were laid, then was also laid the foundation of the Sabbath. I was shown that if the true Sabbath had been kept, there would never have been an infidel

or an atheist. The observance of the Sabbath would have preserved the world from idolatry.

The fourth commandment has been trampled upon, therefore we are called upon to repair the breach in the law and plead for the desecrated Sabbath. The man of sin, who exalted himself above God and thought to change times and laws, brought about the change of the Sabbath from the seventh to the first day of the week. In doing this he made a breach in the law of God. Just prior to the great day of God, a message is sent forth to warn the people to come back to their allegiance to the law of God, which antichrist has broken down. Attention must be called to the breach in the law, by precept and example.

I was shown that the precious promises of Isaiah 58:12–14 apply to those who labor for the restoration of the true Sabbath.

I was shown that the third angel proclaiming the commandments of God and the faith of Jesus, represents the people who receive this message, and raise the voice of warning to the world to keep the commandments of God and His law as the apple of the eye; and that in response to this warning, many would embrace the Sabbath of the Lord.[1] (More about the warning of the third angel in Chapter 28.)

The verses in Isaiah, which Ellen White referred to, are these:

Those from among you
Shall build the old waste places;
You shall raise up the foundations of many generations;
And you shall be called the Repairer of the Breach,
The Restorer of Streets to Dwell In.

"If you turn away your foot from the Sabbath,
From doing your pleasure on My holy day,
And call the Sabbath a delight,

The holy day of the LORD honorable,
And shall honor Him, not doing your own ways,
Nor finding your own pleasure,
Nor speaking your own words,
Then you shall delight yourself in the LORD;
And I will cause you to ride on the high hills of the earth,
And feed you with the heritage of Jacob your father.
The mouth of the LORD has spoken."

The Ten Commandments are a wall of protection and there has been a "breach" in the wall. God has called us to be a "Repairer of the Breach" (Isaiah 58:12). In the Book of Revelation, three angels (messengers) give the last warning to the inhabitants of the entire earth just prior to the return of Jesus. In Revelation 14, God contrasts those who will be "tormented with fire and brimstone" with those "who keep the commandments of God and the faith of Jesus." Keeping Sunday, the first day of the week, in place of the seventh-day Sabbath has been a long-held tradition, but a tradition is still only a tradition no matter how long it has been kept. Jesus warned us about replacing a commandment of God with a tradition of men (Matthew 15:3–7). About 600 years before Jesus became man, the prophet Daniel prophesied that someone would "intend (or try, NIV) to change times and law" (Daniel 7:25). That prophesy came true early in the Christian Church.

I have learned that God loves us and that it is always best to do what He says. Jesus often prefaced His remarks with "it is written" as He did when tempted by the devil to change stones into bread. When tempted, Jesus said, "It is written, 'Man shall not live by bread alone, but by every word that proceeds from the mouth of God'" (Matthew 4:4). In giving that answer, Jesus was quoting the "word of God" from Deuteronomy 8:3.

Would you like to be blessed? Jesus told us how. He said, "Blessed are those who hear the word of God and keep it" (Luke 11:28).

It is not a good idea to use our own judgment if it contradicts God's word. Proverbs 14:12 warns us: "There is a way that seems right to a man, but its end is the way of death." It may seem that it makes no difference what day we keep, but there is no safety in going against God's command, especially one that He spoke out loud and wrote on stone with His own finger.

1. White, E. G. *Life Sketches of Ellen White*. 1915. Pacific Press Publishing Association, Boise, Idaho, 95, 96.

Chapter 25

Climate Change, Natural Disasters, and the Coming of Jesus

For nation will rise against nation, and kingdom against kingdom. And there will be famines, pestilences, and earthquakes in various places. - Matthew 24:7

Once a year in June, Conservation District employees in Washington State converge at the Sleeping Lady resort in Leavenworth for three days of training. We can choose from a variety of concurrent courses. In 2016, a new course was added to the list—Climate Change. Conservation Districts across the country are now investigating ways to adapt to and/or mitigate the effects of a changing climate.

Things Are Warming Up

The June–August 2019 average temperature across global land and ocean surfaces was the second highest average temperature for that three-month period since 1880. The highest three-month average occurred in 2016. The five warmest June–August periods have occurred within the last five years.[1]

The global land and ocean surface temperature for the three-month period has increased at an average rate of 0.13 degrees Fahrenheit per decade since 1880. Since 1981, the average rate of increase has more than doubled (0.32 degrees Fahrenheit per decade). The highest and second highest average sea surface temperature occurred in 2016 and 2019.[1]

In 2015, an anomaly of high temperature surface-water appeared off the West Coast from Alaska to Mexico.[2] This huge expanse of warm water, approaching seven degrees Fahrenheit above average, was nicknamed "the Blob." The warmer water resulted in the largest harmful algal bloom ever recorded on the West Coast, which shut down crabbing and clamming for months. It caused lesser quality food to be available for young salmon, which contributed to low salmon returns. And it resulted in the stranding of young sea lions on California beaches.

In September 2019, as another expanse of warm water, similar in size to "the Blob," was forming off the West Coast. Cisco Werner, NOAA Fisheries Director of Scientific Programs and Chief Science Advisor said, "We learned with 'the Blob' and similar events worldwide that what used to be unexpected is becoming *more common*" (emphasis mine).[2]

Extreme Weather—More Intense and More Frequent

In November 2018, Volume II of the U.S. Climate Change Report was released. This assessment was compiled by the U.S. Global Change Research Program, a consortium of 13 federal agencies with over 300 leading scientists. Soon after its release, David Reidmiller, Director of the National Climate Assessment told reporters, "Extreme weather events are expected to be *more intense* and *more frequent* in a warming world" (emphasis mine).[3]

Three days before Jesus was crucified, the disciples asked Him, "'What will be the sign of Your coming, and of the end of the age?' And Jesus answered and said to them: 'Take heed that no one deceives you. For many will come in My name, saying, 'I am the Christ,' and will deceive many. And you will hear of wars and rumors of wars. See that you are not troubled; for all these things must come to pass, but the end is not yet. For nation will rise against nation, and kingdom against kingdom. And there will be famines, pestilences, and earthquakes in various places. All these are the beginning of sorrows'" (Matthew 24:3–8).

The New International Version as well as several other translations renders the last sentence, "All these are the beginning of *birth pains*" (my emphasis). Birth pains or labor contractions start mild and are far apart, but as birth approaches, they become stronger and closer together. This seems to fit what our country as well as the rest of the world has been experiencing with natural disasters becoming *more intense* and *more frequent*. It also fits the prediction made by David Reidmiller of extreme weather events becoming *"more intense* and *more frequent* in a warming world"* (my emphasis).

In her book *The Great Controversy*,[4] Ellen White made an interesting statement regarding natural disasters:

> Satan works through the elements also to garner his harvest of unprepared souls. He has studied the secrets of the laboratories of nature, and he uses all his power to control the elements as far as God allows. ...
>
> Even now he is at work. In accidents and calamities by sea and by land, in great *conflagrations*, in fierce *tornadoes* and terrific *hailstorms*, in *tempests*, *floods*, *cyclones*, *tidal waves*, and *earthquakes*, in every place and in a thousand forms, Satan is exercising his power. He sweeps away the ripening harvest, and famine and distress follow. He imparts to the air a deadly taint, and thousands perish by the pestilence. These visitations are to become more and more *frequent* and *disastrous* (emphasis mine).

Ellen White goes on to say that the blame for these natural disasters will be placed on those who continue to observe the Bible Sabbath, and that eventually "even in free America, rulers and legislators, *in order to secure public favor, will yield to the popular demand* for a law enforcing Sunday observance" (emphasis mine).[4]

Climate Change and Sunday Rest

Momentum has been building globally to do something about climate change. In September 2019, three significant events took place. Millions of mostly young people rallied in cities across the globe to *demand that their leaders pass laws* that will curb global warming. The United Nations conducted a three-day summit to address climate change. And Pope Francis announced an invitation to representatives from various religions, NGOs, academia, and cultural and political leaders to come to Rome on May 14, 2020 to a Global Education Alliance.[6] The pope stated that the alliance is "to shape the future of humanity by forming mature individuals who can overcome division and care for our common home."

In his opening remarks before giving his invitation to come to Rome, Pope Francis referenced his encyclical *Laudato Si: On Care For Our Common Home,*[5] given five years earlier. In it, Pope Francis critiqued the degradation of the earth's soil, water, and air. He stated, "A very solid scientific consensus indicates that we are presently witnessing a disturbing warming of the climatic system. In recent decades this warming has been accompanied by a constant rise in the sea level and, it would appear, by an increase of extreme weather events..." (Paragraph 23). In the encyclical's closing paragraphs, Pope Francis emphasized the need for ecological education for all people. And in Paragraph 237, he expressed a need for a Sunday day of rest.

Becoming educated about our environment, taking better care of the earth, having a weekly day of rest—all are good and noble goals. The problem I foresee is the day of rest. It will not be the Sabbath, the day God commanded us to rest (Exodus 20:8-11); it will be Sunday, a day instituted by man.

In the book of Revelation, the final issue leading up to the "battle of that great day of God Almighty...Armageddon" will involve the "kings of the earth and of the whole world" (Revelation 16:14-16). Climate change is a world wide issue and it will require action by all the "kings [leaders] of the earth" to address it. Who is in a better position to lead in this effort than the pope?

In 592 B.C. the prophet Ezekiel, then a captive in Babylon, was given a vision of what was occurring in Jerusalem. He was shown sequentially four abominations, each one more abominable than the previous one and each one having to do with idol worship. Ezekiel described the fourth abomination with these words: "At the door of the temple of the

LORD, between the porch and the altar, were about twenty-five men with their backs toward the temple of the LORD and their faces toward the east, and they were *worshiping the sun* toward the east" (Ezekiel 8:16; emphasis mine). Following this, the people who were sighing and crying over all the abominations were marked on their foreheads and all those without this mark were slain (Ezekiel 9:4–6). This marking on the forehead is symbolic of those who, in the last days, receive the "seal of God" and are not harmed (Revelation 9:4). The alternative is to receive the "mark of the beast" and "drink of the wine of the wrath of God" (Revelation 14:9, 10).

I suspect that the climate change issue is going to lead to another worldwide issue—the "day of rest"—choosing Sunday, an institution of man or the seventh-day Sabbath, a commandment of God. This suspicion is not my wild imagination. It is based on Bible prophecy. About 2,500 years ago in Babylon, God's people were faced with a similar decision. Bow down to a golden image—and break God's second commandment—or die in a fiery furnace. Read Chapter 3 in the book of Daniel to find out what happened.

Choosing the "day of rest"—God's rest day or man's rest day— will be the final test that is coming upon the world. Essentially, it is the same test that Adam and Eve were given: trust God and obey Him or be your own god and do what you think. (See what the wise man Solomon said about this alternative in Proverbs 14:12.) Enormous pressure will be put on Sabbath keepers to yield to Sunday observance. At first they will not be able to "buy or sell" (Revelation 13:17), and when this fails, they will face a death decree (Revelation 13:15).

I encourage you to prayerfully study the Bible—God's inspired word—so that you will be divinely informed to make the right choice. The last chapter of this book contains some recommendations about studying the Bible.

1. Anonymous. 2019. Assessing the Global Climate in August 2019. National Oceanic and Atmospheric Administration, September 16, 2019. https://www.ncei.noaa.gov/news/global-climate-201908

2. Anonymous. 2019. New marine heatwave emerges off West Coast, resembles "the Blob." National Oceanic and Atmospheric Administration, NOAA Fisheries News, September 05, 2019. https://www.fisheries.noaa.gov/feature-story/new-marine-heatwave-emerges-west-coast-resembles-blob?utm_medium=email&utm_source=govdelivery

3. Scott Waldman, E&E News reporter Climatewire: November 23, 2018 at 2:39 PM. https://www.eenews.net/staff/Scott_Waldman

4. White, E. G. 1911. *The Great Controversy.* Review and Herald Publishing Association, Mountain View, California, 589, 590, 592.

5. Pope Francis. 2015. Encyclical letter Laudato Si of the Holy Father Francis on care for our common home. http://w2.vatican.va/content/francesco/en/encyclicals/documents/papa-francesco_20150524_enciclica-laudato-si.html

6. Pope Francis. 2019. Pope Francis launches Global Education Alliance. Vatican News, Vatican Radio, 9/20/19. https://www.vaticannews.va/en/pope/news/2019-09/pope-francis-video-message-global-educational-alliance.html

Chapter 26

Coronavirus—Another Sign of the Times

For nation will rise against nation, and kingdom against kingdom. And there will be famines, pestilences, and earthquakes in various places. - Matthew 24:7

In March 2020, as this book was being published, another sign of the times was emerging—a coronavirus known as COVID-19. COVID-19 has largely displaced Climate Change as a hot topic in the news.

In May 2020, as I write this new chapter for the second edition of this book, my life along with the lives of most everyone else has changed drastically in a very short time. I no longer work at the office. I work from home now. Instead of meeting around a table, I attend Zoom meetings. Before entering a store, I don a mask. I no longer greet people with a handshake and am careful to stay at least six feet from everyone. My bank lobby is closed, and I now make deposits by iPhone.

Life in the entire world has changed since COVID-19 made its appearance in Wuhan, China and quickly spread throughout the world. As of this writing, COVID-19 has claimed the lives of 312,000 people of whom 87,000 were from the United States.[1] Millions of people are out of work in the Unites States and other countries. Governments are doing a balancing act between saving the economy and keeping people safe.

Pestilence was one of the signs Jesus spoke of to make us aware when His return is near. Jesus said, "For nation will rise against nation, and kingdom against kingdom. And there will be famines, pestilences, and earthquakes in various places" (Matthew 24:7). COVID-19 is a fulfillment of that prophecy.

Another Sign

Famine, another sign of the nearness of Jesus' return, often accompanies pestilence. In April 2020, a consortium of 16 organizations released the *Global Report on Food Crisis 2020*.[2] The authors assessed situations of food insecurity around the world. In 1919, prior to the spread of COVID-19, 135 million people across 55 countries and territories were classified as being in "crisis." Crisis is defined as being acutely insecure of obtaining food. Another 183 million were classified as "stressed" and were at risk of slipping into crisis if confronted by additional stress. The authors projected that the additional stress caused by COVID-19 could increase the number of people in crisis to 265 million by the end of 2020.

Another Pestilence

In early 2020, another kind of pestilence occurred in several countries in East Africa and South Asia. Hundreds of billions of locusts, a gregarious form of grasshoppers, ravaged croplands. The Food and Agriculture Organization estimated that a swarm of locusts covering one square kilometer of land can consume in one day the equivalent amount of food that would feed 35,000 humans. Making matters worse, they predicted that warming temperatures due to Climate Change will benefit the locusts.[3]

Global Response

In the same way that Climate Change is a world-wide issue requiring world leadership, so it is with COVID-19. In a March 2020 interview, Pope Francis linked COVID-19 with our failure to address Climate Change.

When asked to comment on the COVID-19 pandemic, Pope Francis said, "We did not respond to the partial catastrophes. Who now speaks of the fires in Australia, or remembers that 18 months ago a boat could cross the North Pole because the glaciers had all melted? Who speaks of the floods? I don't know if these are the revenge of nature, but they are certainly nature's responses."[4]

On April 22, 2020, the 50th anniversary of the first Earth day, Pope Francis made an impassioned plea for the protection of the environment. He said that the coronavirus pandemic had shown that some challenges had to be met with a global response.[5]

Who is in a better position to lead a global response than the pope? As mentioned in the previous chapter, Pope Francis invited religious, academic, NGO, cultural, and political leaders to Rome on May 14, 2020 to address Climate Change. Due to COVID-19, the meeting has been postponed until October 2020. Since Pope Francis has already suggested that COVID-19 is "nature's response" to Climate Change, it would not be surprising that both Climate Change and COVID-19 are on the agenda in October. And it will not be surprising to me that part of the answer to both problems will be observing a "day of rest." But it will not be God's day of rest.

1. World Health Organization Coronavirus Disease (COVID-19) Dashboard. https://covid19.who.int/?gclid=EAIaIQobChMIgpSc2_O96QIV9T6tB h1bhAA6EAAYASAAEgL5qvD_BwE

2. GRFC 2020. Global report on food crises: Joint analyses for better decisions. Global Network Against Food Crises; Food Security Information Network. https://www.fsinplatform.org/sites/default/files/resources/files/GRFC_2 020_ONLINE_200420.pdf

3. Simon, M. 2020. The terrifying science behind the locust plagues of Africa. Science 02- 05-2020. https://www.wired.com/story/the-terrifying-science-behind-the-locust-plagues-of-africa/

4. Ivereigh, A. 2020. Pope Francis says pandemic can be a 'place of conversion.' The Tablet, April 8, 2020. https://www.thetablet.co.uk/features/2/17845/pope-francis-says-pandemic-can-be-a-place-of-conversion-

5. Pullella, P. 2020. On earth day, Pope says nature will not forgive

our trespasses. U.S. News, April 22, 2020. https://www.usnews.com/news/world/articles/2020-04-22/on-earth-day-pope-says-nature-will-not-forgive-our-trespasses

Chapter 27
The Sure Word of Prophecy

Surely the Lord God does nothing, unless He reveals His secret to His
servants the prophets. - Amos 3:7

The increase in intensity and frequency of natural disasters is not the only way we know that Jesus' coming is near. We have the sure word of prophecy. The apostle Peter wrote: "And so we have the prophetic word confirmed, which you do well to heed as a light that shines in a dark place, until the day dawns and the morning star [Jesus] rises in your hearts; knowing this first, that no prophecy of Scripture is of any private interpretation, for prophecy never came by the will of man, but holy men of God spoke as they were moved by the Holy Spirit" (2 Peter 1:19–21).

It is the fulfillment of prophecy that gives us overwhelming confidence in the veracity of the Bible—that its authors were "moved by the Holy Spirit." Numerous prophecies made in the Old Testament were accurately fulfilled in the New Testament. For instance: Jesus would be born in Bethlehem to a virgin; He would be betrayed by a friend; He would be sold for thirty pieces of silver; He would be rejected by His own people; He would be spat upon, smitten, scorned, and mocked. (See Appendix B to see how these prophecies were fulfilled.)

Time of the End

Let's look at a prophecy in the book of Daniel that clearly shows that we are living in the *time of the end*. The angel said to Daniel, "But you, Daniel, shut up the words, and seal the book until the *time of the end*;

many shall run to and fro, and knowledge shall increase" (Daniel 12:4; emphasis mine). Much of the book of Daniel has been understood for centuries, but not all of the book—particularly the prophecy of Daniel 8:14: "For two thousand three hundred days; then the sanctuary shall be cleansed."

In the early1800s the Holy Spirit enlightened the minds of people independently in different parts of the world for a more complete understanding of the Book of Daniel. In the United States one such person was William Miller, a farmer in upstate New York. After years of prayerful study, Miller began understanding the 2300-day prophecy. In Daniel 9:25 he found that the prophecy started at the "command to restore and build Jerusalem." In the Book of Ezra (7:8, 13) he found that Persian King Artaxerxes gave this command in the seventh year of his reign, which occurred in 457 BC. Based on the principle that one day of prophetic time represents one year (Ezekiel 4:6; Numbers 14:34), Miller added 2300 years to 457 BC and arrived at 1843. When he discovered that there is only 1 year from 1 BC to AD 1, not 2 years, he corrected the date to 1844.

In Miller's day it was a common belief that the cleansing of the sanctuary referred to the cleansing of the earth with fire when Jesus returned. The belief that Jesus was soon to return spread like wildfire throughout the Northeastern United States and in other parts of the world and many prepared to meet Jesus. Believers in the soon return of Jesus became known as Millerites.

Further study pinpointed the exact date of Jesus' expected return. They reasoned from the Scriptures that the cleansing of the sanctuary took place on the Day of Atonement (Yom Kippur) and the Day of Atonement came on the tenth day of the seventh Jewish month. In 1844 the Day of Atonement fell on October 22.

When Jesus did not return on October 22, 1844, the Millerites were bitterly disappointed. Many gave up their faith, but some, feeling that the Holy Spirit had led them this far, prayed for enlightenment.

God answered their prayers. They learned that they had the date right, but the event wrong. God led them to the book of Hebrews for the correct understanding of the "cleansing of the sanctuary." They discovered that on October 22, 1844, Jesus, our High Priest, entered the Most Holy Place of the sanctuary in Heaven to begin a work of atonement.

The work of atonement includes judgment. Jesus said, "And behold, I am coming quickly, and My reward is with Me, to give to every one according to his work" (Revelation 22:12). In Chapter 19, we saw that only the "saved" will be resurrected when Jesus returns; the "lost" are resurrected 1000 years later. Thus, a judgment is necessary *before* Jesus returns.

Not long ago I studied this prophecy with a friend. Jim said, "How do we know what is happening in Heaven since we can't see it."

I replied, "That is true; we cannot see it. But there are a lot of things I have not seen, but believe. I have not seen Jesus walking on water (Matthew 14:25) or calming the wind (Mark 4:39), and I have not seen the place in Heaven Jesus went to prepare for us (John 14:2), but I believe it."

We cannot "see" the judgment taking place in Heaven. We need to see it through the "eyes of faith," but it is not blind faith.

What gives credence to the 1844 date is the precise fulfillment of other events that took place in the first 490 years of the 2300-year prophecy (Daniel 9:24-27). In the last seven years of the 490 years, three events were prophesied (see chart below):

1.   At the beginning of the last seven years the Messiah was to come.

2.   In the middle of the week He was to be cut off (die) and bring an end to sacrifice.

3.   He was to confirm the gospel covenant during the last seven years.

These three events were fulfilled exactly on time:

1.   In AD 27 Jesus, the Messiah, was anointed by the Holy Spirit at His baptism and He began His public work.

2.   Three and one-half years later in AD 31, Jesus was crucified.

3.   From AD 27 to AD 34 the gospel covenant was preached to the Jews, first by Jesus and then by the disciples. The stoning of Stephen in AD 34 marked the beginning of all-out persecution of the Christians. At this time the disciples dispersed and began taking the gospel to the Gentiles.

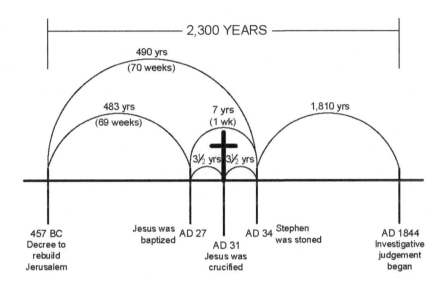

Daniel was told to "seal up the book until the *time of the end*" (Daniel 12:4; emphasis mine). The unsealing of the 2300-year prophecy, indicating that judgment began in 1844, marked the beginning of the *time of the end*. We are now living in the time of the end!

The Most Important Book

Of all the books in the world—about 130 million according to Google—the Bible is the most important because it is inspired by God and tells us how to have eternal life. "All Scripture is given by inspiration of God, and is profitable for doctrine, for reproof, for correction, for instruction in righteousness" (2 Timothy 3:16).

In every age the Bible contains truth that is especially important for that particular time. For example, about 4,500 years ago, when Noah was building the ark, it was important to know that it was going to rain and that one's survival depended upon hearing and acting upon God's word spoken through His prophet Noah. It was not enough to *hear* what Noah was saying. If you did not *enter the ark* you perished in the flood.

In the book *Patriarchs and Prophets*,[1] Ellen White said that "some people were deeply convicted, and would have heeded the words of warning; but there were so many to jest and ridicule, that they partook of the same spirit, [and] resisted the invitations of mercy." They sided with the majority and perished in the flood. God's true followers have always been in the minority; there is no safety in numbers. There is also no safety in automatically believing what pastors, priests, and popes say. It was the religious leaders who had Jesus crucified! One's eternal destiny is too important to leave to someone else. Prayerfully read the Bible for yourself.

As it was important in Noah's day, it is equally important today to know, understand, and *put into practice* what God has revealed to us in the books of Daniel and Revelation. Even a cursory glance at these books tells us they were written for the people living in the *time of the end.*

Some people say, "the Book of Revelation is just too hard to understand" or "it's too scary."

But look at the first three verses: "The *Revelation of Jesus Christ,* which God gave Him to show His servants—things which must shortly take place. And He sent and signified it [put it in symbols] by His angel to His servant John, who bore witness to the word of God, and to the testimony of Jesus Christ, to all things that he saw. *Blessed* is he who *reads* and those who *hear* the words of this prophecy, and *keep* those things which are written in it; for the time is near" (Revelation 1:1–3; emphasis mine).

To "read" is to gain knowledge. To "hear" is to understand it. And to "keep" is to put it into practice. Be like the *wise man* that built on the Rock and put God's word into practice! (Matthew 7:24–27).

Distractions

The devil's greatest strategy is distraction, keeping us occupied with the things of this world. Paul gave us good advice: "While we do not look at the things which are seen, but at the things which are not seen.

For the things which are seen are temporary, but the things which are not seen are eternal" (2 Corinthians 4:18). The disciple John said, "For all that is in the world—the lust of the flesh, the lust of the eyes, and the pride of life—is not of the Father but is of the world. And the world is passing away, and the lust of it; but he who *does the will* of God abides forever" (1 John 2:16, 17). Jesus said, "But seek first the kingdom of God and His righteousness, and all these things shall be added to you" (Matthew 6:33). What is more important—the trinkets of this world or your eternal life?

Doers of the Word

Thankfully, we do not have to start at the beginning to interpret the symbols in Daniel and Revelation. We can learn from others (Chapter 30 has some helpful resources). Before you study and as you study, ask God for the Holy Spirit, the Spirit of truth, to give you knowledge and understanding. God will guide you. Jesus said that the Spirit of Truth will guide us into all truth and that He will tell us things to come (John 16:13). Pray for the courage to put into practice what the Spirit reveals to you even if you are in the minority, the only one in your neighborhood or even the only one in your family.

Remember what Jesus said, "Everyone who has left houses or brothers or sisters or father or mother or wife or children or lands, for My name's sake, shall receive a hundredfold, and inherit eternal life" (Matthew 19:29).

Genuine Christians are the *doers* of God's word! We are fortunate—probably by God's design—that the time of the end is occurring in the age of communication. Many will learn in a short time what others have taken a lifetime to learn.

1. White, E. G. 1958. *Patriarchs and Prophets*. Review and Herald Publishing Association, Mountain View, California, 95.

Chapter 28
The Sanctuary—God's Restoration Plan in Symbols

Your way, O God, is in the sanctuary; Who is so great a God as our God?
- Psalm 77:13

Have you ever wondered, if God is love and all powerful, why does He allow suffering, death, and injustice to continue? It is almost 2,000 years since Jesus declared, "It is finished!" (John 19:30). We know that the tomb did not hold Jesus and that He ascended to Heaven forty days after His resurrection (Acts 1:9). What has Jesus been doing for the past 2,000 years? Why do sin and suffering continue? Why do the rich get richer and the poor get poorer?

The psalmist Asaph asked these same questions (Psalm 73:16, 17). He found the answer in the sanctuary service and we can too.

Symbols of God's Restoration Plan

When God gave Moses the Ten Commandments on Mount Sinai, he also gave him detailed instructions on building a sanctuary (Exodus 25–28). This sanctuary was a pattern or scale model of the sanctuary in Heaven (Hebrews 8:1–5).

The sanctuary consisted of three main divisions (see figure):

1. The Courtyard,
2. The Holy Place
3. The Most Holy Place

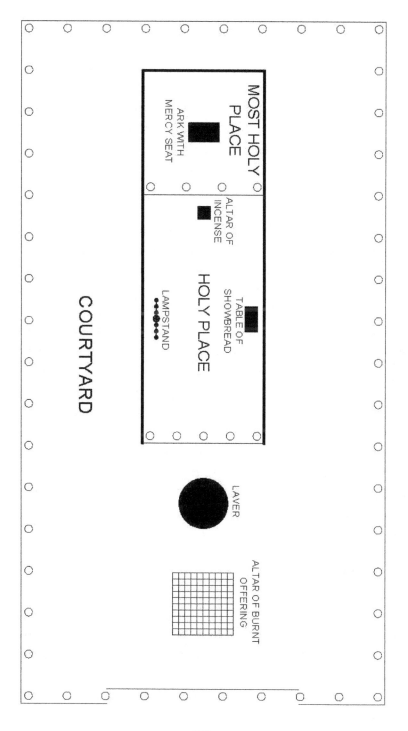

In each division were articles of furniture that symbolized God's restoration plan (see diagram).

The courtyard with its *single* entrance came first. The entrance represents Jesus who said, "I am the door. If anyone enters by Me, he will be saved" (John 10:9). He also said, "I am the way, the truth, and the life. No one comes to the Father except through Me" (John 14:6).

Inside the courtyard was the bronze altar of burnt offering. A sinner brought a sacrificial animal, often a lamb, to the courtyard. The sinner placed his hands on the head of the lamb and confessed his sins. He then cut the lamb's throat and the priest caught the blood in a basin. The priest placed some blood on the horns projecting from the four corners of the bronze altar and poured the remainder at the base of the altar. He then burned the fat of the lamb on the altar.

For some sin offerings the priest took some blood into the Holy Place and sprinkled it before the veil, behind which was the ark containing the Ten Commandments. Symbolically, the sins were transferred from the sinner, to the innocent lamb, to the blood, to the priest, and lastly to the sanctuary. Thus, the sins were transferred from the sinner to the sanctuary.

The innocent lamb died in place of the sinner. Jesus, the Lamb of God, bore our sins and died in our place (John 1:29; 1 Peter 2:24).

A bronze laver containing water stood between the altar of burnt offering and the Holy Place. The priest washed his hands and feet before entering and leaving the Holy Place. Washing in the laver represents cleansing and symbolizes baptism (Titus 3:5). We are cleansed by the blood of Jesus (1 John 1:7).

The Holy Place

Next in line is the Holy Place, which contains three articles of furniture. On the right or north side was the table of showbread. Jesus said, "I am the bread of Life" (John 6:48). Jesus is our Sustainer. His words provide spiritual nourishment. Jeremiah said, "Your words were found, and I ate them" (Jeremiah 15:16).

On the left or south side was the lampstand. Jesus said, "I am the light of the world" (John 8:12). Jesus is our enlightenment. He told us to let our light shine and to be the light of the world (Matthew 5:14, 16).

The third article of furniture in the Holy Place was the altar of incense. The incense is the fragrance of the merit of Christ's righteousness that is mingled with our prayers. Jesus entered the Holy Place of the sanctuary in Heaven forty days after He rose from the dead. There He mediates between us and God the Father.

As discussed in the previous chapter, on October 22, 1844 Jesus moved from the Holy Place to the Most Holy Place where, in addition to interceding for us, He began the work of atonement.

The Most Holy Place

In the Most Holy Place was a precious chest of wood called the ark. Above the ark and forming its cover was the mercy seat. Two golden cherubim, one on each side of the ark, covered the mercy seat with their wings. Before Lucifer led the rebellion in Heaven, he was one of the covering cherubim (Ezekiel 28:14).

The Mercy Seat

On the day of atonement, when the high priest entered the Most Holy Place, he sprinkled the mercy seat with the blood of a bull for his own sins and with the blood of the Lord's goat for the sins of the people. Today in Heaven, Jesus presents His own blood before the mercy seat as He intercedes for us.

The Ark

Inside the sacred ark were the Ten Commandments, Aaron's rod, and a golden pot of manna. The Book of the Law was "beside" or "in the side of" (KJV) the ark. (Deuteronomy 31:26).

The Ten Commandments

The Ten Commandments were inscribed by God's finger on two tables of stone: the first four commandments on one table and the last six on the other. The penalty for breaking God's law is death. We have all broken God's law, but we need not despair for Jesus died for us and fulfilled the law for us. "When, through faith in Jesus Christ, man does according to the very best of his ability, and seeks to keep the way of the Lord by obedience to the Ten Commandments, the perfection of Christ is imputed to cover the transgression of the repentant and obedient soul."[1] "There is therefore now no condemnation to those who are in Christ Jesus, who do not walk according to the flesh, but according to the Spirit" (Romans 8:1).

Manna

The manna, which came down from Heaven to sustain life during the Israelites' forty years in the wilderness, represented Jesus. Jesus came down from Heaven and gave His life to the world (John 6:31–33). The Ten Commandments were in effect prior to God giving them to Moses. This is evident from the account of the manna in the wilderness.

The Israelites were told to gather twice as much manna on the sixth day of the week as on the five preceding days. They were not to gather manna on the Sabbath because it was a day of rest. They were to gather an extra portion on the sixth day to eat on the Sabbath. If they tried to save some manna gathered on any other day than the Sabbath, it would have worms and stink on the next day. Some disobeyed and looked for manna on the Sabbath, but found none. "And the Lord said to Moses, 'How long do you refuse to keep my commandments and my laws?'" (Exodus 16:28). This experience occurred prior to God giving the Ten Commandments to Moses.

Aaron's Rod

Aaron's rod, which produced buds, blossoms, and almonds overnight, was preserved in the ark as a reminder of the deadly effects of pride, envy, and self-exaltation. These sins led Korah to covet Moses' position. As a result, Korah, his family, and about 15,000 followers died in the rebellion (Numbers 16). The same sins led to the downfall of Lucifer and one-third of his angel-followers in Heaven. Ultimately, it will lead to the death of many of his followers on earth. (Isaiah 14:12–15).

After the death of Korah and his followers, God told each of the leaders of the twelve tribes of Israel to bring a rod with their name written on it. Moses then placed the rods in the tabernacle. The next day, the rod of Aaron of the house of Levi, bore buds, blossoms, and ripe almonds. God instructed Moses to put Aaron's rod in the tabernacle as a perpetual reminder of the consequence of rebellion (Numbers 17).

The Book of the Law

The Book of the Law was written on a scroll by Moses as God directed him. It contained testimonies, statutes and judgments (Deuteronomy 5:44). Unlike the Ten-Commandment-Law, written by God on stone and placed inside the ark, the book of the law was placed beside the ark. Referred to as the ceremonial law, the book of the law contained directions regarding the sacrificial service, which pointed forward to the sacrifice of Jesus. When Jesus died on the cross, the veil between the Holy Place and the Most Holy Place was torn from top to bottom, signifying the end of the sacrificial system (Matthew 27:51). It was this sacrificial law that the apostle Paul said was nailed to the cross (Colossians 2:14).

Many Christians mistakenly believe that the Ten-Commandment-Law was nailed to the cross and that the Ten Commandments are no longer binding. It is true that we are saved by God's grace and not by keeping the law, but to say the Ten Commandments are no longer binding is to say it is all right to steal, kill, commit adultery, etc.

Paul pronounced the Ten-Commandment-Law "holy and just and good" (Romans 7:12). David wrote, "The law of the LORD is perfect, converting the soul" (Psalms 19:7). Jesus said, "Do not think that I came to destroy the Law or the Prophets. I did not come to destroy but to fulfill. For assuredly, I say to you, till heaven and earth pass away, one jot or one tittle will by no means pass from the law till all is fulfilled" (Matthew 5:17, 18). In His sermon on the mount, Jesus *magnified* the law. He taught that obeying the law went *beyond* keeping the letter of the law. He said that becoming angry without cause is breaking the commandment not to murder (Matthew 5:21, 22) and lusting at a woman is breaking the commandment not to commit adultery (Matthew 5:27, 28). Jesus demonstrated what a life looks like when the commandments are written on the heart.

What exactly did Paul mean when he wrote to the Galatians that we are not "under law" (Galatians 5:18)? He meant that we are not saved by keeping the law (i.e., by good works). As Paul wrote to the Ephesians, we are saved by grace through faith (Ephesians 2:8). This is good news because we have all failed to keep the law. However, being saved by grace does not do away with the law that is holy, just, and good and that is the foundation of God's government.

Atonement and Judgment

The work of atonement requires a work of judgment. It is true that Jesus died for the sins of the whole world. His sacrifice, represented by the altar of burnt offering in the courtyard, was accomplished for every single person whoever lived. Sadly however, not everyone who takes the name of Christian is a genuine Christian. In the Most Holy Place of the heavenly sanctuary, Jesus is now conducting the judgment. He is checking wedding garments (Matthew 22:1–14), separating good fish from bad fish (Matthew 13:47–50), and sheep from goats (Matthew 25:32, 33).

In *The Desire of Ages*,[2] Ellen White wrote, "Many take it for granted that they are Christians, simply because they subscribe to certain theological tenets. But they have not brought the truth into practical life." In *Early Writings*[3] she wrote, "Very many who profess to be Christians have not known God. The natural heart has not been changed, and the carnal mind remains at enmity with God. They are Satan's faithful servants, notwithstanding they have assumed another name."

Jesus said, "Not everyone who says to Me, 'Lord, Lord,' shall enter the kingdom of heaven, but he who does the will of My Father in heaven. Many will say to Me in that day, 'Lord, Lord, have we not prophesied in Your name, cast out demons in Your name, and done many wonders in Your name?' And then I will declare to them, 'I never knew you; depart from Me, you who practice lawlessness!'" (Matthew 7:21–23).

Thus, the blood of the atonement is applied only to genuine Christians. The Bible says that we are not saved by our works (Ephesians

2:8), but it also says that we are judged by them, "by the things which were written in the books" (Revelation 20:12; Daniel 7:10).

When the investigative judgment is finished, our opportunity to repent of our sins and accept Jesus as our Lord and Savior will be over. Jesus will pronounce the solemn words, "He who is unjust, let him be unjust still; he who is filthy, let him be filthy still; he who is righteous, let him be righteous still; he who is holy, let him be holy still" (Revelation 22:11). Then Jesus will say, "Behold, I am coming quickly, and My reward is with Me, to give to every one according to his work" (Revelation 22:12).

The judgment must take place before Jesus returns because only the saved are resurrected at that time; the rest of the dead, the lost, remain in the grave for another 1,000 years (Revelation 20:5; see Chapter 19).

At the return of Jesus, the saved, both those alive and those who are resurrected, receive their glorified, immortal bodies (1 Thessalonians 4:16, 17; 1 Corinthians 15:53). At this time the restoration of God's people is complete. They are restored to the image of God!

Cleansing the Sanctuary

We have seen how sins were symbolically transferred from the sinner to the sacrificial animal, to the blood, to the priest, and to the sanctuary. Figuratively speaking, sins have been accumulating in the sanctuary for a long time and it is in need of cleansing.

But how is the sanctuary cleansed? The Old Testament model gives us the answer. Once a year on the Day of Atonement, known as Yom Kippur, the high priest entered the Most Holy Place for the cleansing ceremony. Two goats were brought to the door of the sanctuary and lots were cast for them—one lot for the Lord, and the other lot for the scapegoat. The Lord's goat was slain as a sin offering for the people. The high priest sprinkled its blood on the mercy seat over the Ten Commandments and on the altar of incense before the veil.

The high priest laid both his hands on the head of the live goat and confessed all the sins of the people. The goat, bearing all the sins of the people, was then taken into an uninhabited land by a man specially chosen for the task. Thus, the sins, which had been transferred to the sanctuary through the blood of the sacrificial animals, were born by the high priest, transferred to the scapegoat, and removed from the sanctuary. The sanctuary was now cleansed of sin.

Before returning to camp, the man was required to wash himself and his clothing. The whole ceremony was to impress the people with the holiness of God and His abhorrence of sin. On the Day of Atonement, the people were to spend the day in solemn humiliation before God, with prayer, fasting, and deep searching of heart.

This ceremonial cleansing of the sanctuary, repeated annually in the earthly sanctuary, represents what is occurring now in the sanctuary in Heaven. At the end of the 2300 years on October 22, 1844, Jesus our High Priest entered the Most Holy Place in the heavenly sanctuary. At that time He began examining the books of record to determine who, through repentance of sin and faith in His cleansing blood, are entitled to the benefits of the atonement. This investigative judgment is preliminary to the removal of sins from the sanctuary.

When the judgment is completed, Jesus will return for his people, those who are sleeping and those who are alive. They will meet Jesus in the air (1 Thessalonians 4:17) and go to Heaven to the place He has prepared for us (John 14:2, 3). As discussed in Chapter 19, at this time there are no humans left alive on earth. All the sins of the truly penitent are placed upon the scapegoat Satan and he is "bound for a thousand years" to an uninhabited land (Revelation 20:2).

At the close of the thousand years, Jesus returns with all His people and the City of New Jerusalem. The resurrection of the lost occurs. Satan marshals them together and attempts to capture New Jerusalem. "And they went up on the breadth of the earth, and compassed the camp of the saints about, and the beloved city: and fire came down from God out of heaven, and devoured them. And the devil that deceived them was cast into the lake of fire" (Revelation 20:9, 10). Satan comes to his end "and shall be no more forever" (Ezekiel 28:19).

The New Earth

Then Jesus will create the New Earth (Revelation 21:1), and the meek in their immortal, glorified bodies will collect their inheritance

(Matthew 5:5; 1 Corinthians 15:51–54). When this happens, restoration is complete! Men and women in their immortal, glorified bodies will have dominion over the New Earth. They will plant vineyards and till the soil now free of thorns and thistles. They will build country houses to live in when they are not staying in the Holy City, New Jerusalem. And, best of all, they will see God and talk to Him face to face! Praise our wonderful God, wonderful Savior, and wonderful Holy Spirit!

After "walking" through the sanctuary, we now understand that there is more to God's restoration plan than the substitutionary death of Jesus, represented by the altar of burnt offering in the courtyard.

God's Restoration Plan

God's Restoration Plan has three phases:

1. Justification—The Courtyard
2. Sanctification—The Holy Place
3. Glorification—The Most Holy Place

Justification occurs in the courtyard when we accept the sacrifice of Jesus and are baptized. Here Christ's righteousness is legally imputed to us and we are delivered from the penalty of sin—the second death.

Sanctification occurs in the Holy Place. It is here where we grow spiritually becoming more like Jesus day by day as we feed on the word of God, pray to our Father, and let our light shine. Here we are delivered from the power of sin.

Glorification occurs in the Most Holy Place. It is in this phase that our mortal, corruptible bodies become immortal and incorruptible and Satan is destroyed forever. Here we are delivered from the presence of sin.

Since 1844, Jesus has been conducting the investigative judgment in the Most Holy Place. When will the judgment be over? When will Jesus come? There is no time prophecy telling us this, but we do have a statement from Ellen White in *Christ's Object Lessons*[4]:

"The fruit of the Spirit is love, joy, peace, longsuffering, gentleness, goodness, faith, meekness, temperance." Gal. 5:22,

23. This fruit can never perish, but will produce after its kind a harvest unto eternal life.

"When the fruit is brought forth, immediately he putteth in the sickle, because the harvest is come" [Mark 4:29, KJV; emphasis mine]. Christ is waiting with longing desire for the manifestation of Himself in His church. When the character of Christ shall be perfectly reproduced in His people, then He will come to claim them as His own.

It is the privilege of every Christian not only to look for but to hasten the coming of our Lord Jesus Christ (2 Peter 3:12, margin). Were all who profess His name bearing fruit to His glory, how quickly the whole world would be sown with the seed of the gospel. Quickly the last great harvest would be ripened, and Christ would come to gather the precious grain.

For Further Study

For a deeper understanding of the "cleansing of the sanctuary," read the chapter, "What is the Sanctuary?" in *The Great Controversy*.[5] You may also watch a video on this important subject by Pastor Stephen Bohr of Secrets Unsealed.[6]

---

1. White, E. G. 1923. *Fundamentals of Christian education.* Southern Publishing Association, Nashville, Tennessee, 135.

2. White, E. G. 1898. *The Desire of Ages,* Pacific Press Publishing Association, Mountain View, California, 309.

3. White, E. G. 1882. *Early Writings.* Review and Herald Publishing Association, Mountain View, California, 274.

4. White, E. G. 1900. *Christ's Object Lessons.* Review and Herald Publishing Association, Washington, DC, 68, 69.

5. White, E. G. 1911. *The Great Controversy.* Review and Herald Publishing Association, Mountain View, California, 409–422.

6. *The Prophecy of the Seventy Weeks: A New Look at the Blessed Hope,* number 5 of a series of 12 videos by Pastor Stephen Bohr of Secrets Unsealed. https://www.youtube.com/watch?v=s0FsHlWW3do.

Chapter 29
The Three Angels' Messages

*Blessed is he who reads and those who hear the words of this prophecy,
and keep those things which are written in it; for the time is near.* -
Revelation 1:3

We are living in the *time of the end*. Very soon Jesus will come to take
His people home. In the story of the ten virgins, the bridegroom came at
midnight (Matthew 25:6). We are living in the eleventh hour of earth's
history. You may be in the eleventh hour of your life and have not yet
accepted Jesus as your Savior. But it is not too late! The door to God's
kingdom is still open. In a parable Jesus told about the kingdom of
Heaven, some laborers did not start working in the vineyard until the
eleventh hour. However, they received the same reward (salvation) as
those who started working early in the morning (Matthew 20:1–16).
This is good news for those of us who squandered a good portion of our
lives!

The door of mercy will soon close on the inhabitants of earth. But
before it closes, God makes a final appeal. This three-part appeal is
known as the "three angels' messages" (Revelation 14:6–11).

The First Angel's Message
"Then I saw another angel flying in the midst of heaven, having the
everlasting gospel to preach to those who dwell on the earth—to every
nation, tribe, tongue, and people— saying with a loud voice, 'Fear God
and give glory to Him, for the hour of His judgment has come; and
worship Him who made heaven and earth, the sea and springs of water'"

(Revelation 14:6, 7).

The Greek word for angel, *aggelos*, can also be translated "messenger." God's people living just before Jesus comes are the three messengers. They proclaim three final messages to the entire world. The first message includes the preaching of the everlasting gospel—salvation through Jesus Christ.

The inhabitants of the earth are told to fear or revere God—"to stand in awe of Him" (Psalm 33:8). Think about this: Jesus, "Who, being in very nature God, did not consider equality with God something to be used to his own advantage; rather, he made himself nothing by taking the very nature of a servant, being made in human likeness [forever]. And being found in appearance as a man, he humbled himself by becoming obedient to death—even death on a cross!" (Philippians 2:6–8, NIV). *Does this not make you stand in awe of the sovereign God of the universe who would do this to save you?*

The Bible repeatedly associates fearing or revering God with His forgiveness and mercy (Psalm 5:7; 33:18; 103:11, 17; 118:4; 130:34; 147:11). When Jesus' mother Mary met her cousin Elizabeth, she sang a song with the words: "His mercy is on those who fear Him" (Luke 1:50).

We are told to give glory to God. Moses asked God to show him His glory. God revealed His character to Moses: merciful, gracious, compassionate, longsuffering, good, truthful, forgiving, and just. (Exodus 33:18, 19; 34:6, 7). We give glory to God when our character is like His—when we live our lives like Jesus lived His life.

Revelation 14:7 says that the "hour of His judgment has come." In the previous chapter we learned that judgment began in 1844 when Jesus entered the Most Holy Place of the Heavenly Sanctuary. Judgment continues almost to the time when Jesus returns. When judgment ends, the door of mercy closes and our fate is sealed. We do not know when this occurs. It is not a matter of *getting* ready; it is a matter of *being* ready. "*Now* is the day of salvation" (2 Corinthians 6:2).

Revelation 14 instructs us to "worship Him who made heaven and earth, the sea and springs of water." This language is very similar to that in the fourth commandment to "Remember the Sabbath day, to keep it holy. ... For in six days the LORD made the heavens and the earth, the sea, and all that is in them, and rested the seventh day" (Exodus 20:8–11).

The "springs of water" refer to the worldwide flood of Noah's day when the "springs of the great deep burst forth" (Genesis 7:11). Noah's warning to avoid destruction is similar to that of the three angels.[1]

The Second Angel's Message

"And another angel followed, saying, 'Babylon is fallen, is fallen, that great city, because she has made all nations drink of the wine of the wrath of her fornication'" (Revelation 14:8).

The great city is Rome. Wine refers to false teachings. Babylon is the apostate church, known as the "little horn" in Daniel that "cast truth down to the ground" and "cast the sanctuary down" (Daniel 8:11, 12). Truths regarding salvation and restoration, symbolized in the sanctuary, were replaced with false teachings: tradition superseding scripture; the elevation of Mary as co-redemtrix; confession made to men instead to God; praying to dead people (saints); purgatory; forever burning hell; indulgences; infant baptism; baptism by sprinkling; and claiming to have changed the fourth commandment.

The mother church is not alone in teaching error. Babylon is the "mother of harlots" (Revelation 17:5). The mother church has many daughter churches that have inherited some of her false teachings.

During the Dark Ages from 538 to 1798, the church used civil government to enforce her beliefs. This illicit relationship of the church and state is called fornication. As the deadly wound is healed (Revelation 13:12), we will again see the church use the power of the state to enforce her beliefs. Civil government will enforce Sunday rest, in opposition to God's true day of rest—the seventh-day Sabbath. When this happens, know that time is *extremely* short; it is *minutes* to midnight. It is time to declare your allegiance to God and to obey His commandment rather than the commandment of men.

We know God has people in Babylon because He is calling them out: "Come out of her *my people*, lest you share in her sins, and lest you receive of her plagues" (Revelation 18:4). God's people will hear His voice and come out.

The Third Angel's Message

"Then a third angel followed them, saying with a loud voice, 'If anyone worships the beast and his image, and receives his mark on his forehead or on his hand, he himself shall also drink of the wine of the wrath of God, which is poured out full strength into the cup of His indignation. He shall be tormented with fire and brimstone in the presence of the holy angels and in the presence of the Lamb. And the smoke of their torment ascends forever and ever; and they have no rest day or night, who worship the beast and his image, and whoever receives the mark of his name'" (Revelation 14: 9–11).

God's worshipers also receive a distinguishing seal on their foreheads. Destroying angels were told not to harm anyone with the seal of God on their foreheads (Revelation 9:4). The Sabbath is the identifying sign or seal of God's people (Ezekiel 20:12; Romans 4:11). God's people enter His Sabbath rest and cease from their works as God did from His (Hebrews 4:10). They cease trying to even *partly* earn their salvation and rest *totally* on the life and death of their Savior Jesus.

The beast power, the apostate church, claims to have changed the day of rest from the seventh day to the first day of the week as a sign of her authority. But in the ark of the covenant in the Most Holy Place of the sanctuary in Heaven are the Ten Commandments, written by the finger of God. They still read: "Remember the Sabbath day, to keep it holy" (Exodus 20:8). Not one word has been changed.

God identifies His people as those who "keep the commandments of God" (Revelation 12:17; 14:12). Wise King Solomon was right when he said, "Fear God, and keep his commandments: for this is the whole duty of man" (Ecclesiastes 12:13, KJV).

The mark or seal on the forehead is not something physical that one can see; it is what we believe in our mind. Paul wrote, "When you believed, you were marked in him with a seal, the promised Holy Spirit" (Ephesians 1:13, NIV).

No one has received the "mark of the beast" yet. However, the day is approaching when the observance of the Sabbath will become a worldwide issue. Sabbath-keepers will receive the blame for the calamities that are occurring in the world with increasing intensity and frequency. Enormous pressure will be put on them to worship on a false sabbath—the first day of the week—and thereby receive the "mark of the beast."

At first, they will not be able to buy or sell and finally they will receive a death sentence (Revelation 13:15, 17). God's people will be severely tested during this time. Jesus warned us: "You will be hated by all for My name's sake."

But Jesus continued, "he who *endures to the end* shall be saved" (Mark 13:13, emphasis mine). Whatever God's people go through, they will not be alone. Just as Jesus was with the three Hebrews in the fiery furnace (Daniel 3:25), so will He be with us. He has promised, "I will never leave you nor forsake you" (Hebrews 13:5). Jesus will deliver His people! (Daniel 12:1).

For additional information on this important subject, read Appendix C.

1. An excellent video, *The Days of Noah*, comparing our day to Noah's day may be obtained here: http://www.lmn.org/catalog/product_info.php/products_id/4954/osCsid/jgbqleepbk0202d2g8dqht4v61

Chapter 30

Science of Salvation—the Everlasting Gospel

For I am not ashamed of the gospel of Christ, for it is the power of God to salvation for everyone who believes, for the Jew first and also for the Greek. - Romans 1:16

In college, I studied the sciences of physics, chemistry, and biology. None of these compare to the science of salvation. The science of salvation is the everlasting gospel, which is the power to save anyone who yields to God's unfailing, unconditional, unmerited love.

In his letter to the Romans, the apostle Paul wrote: "For I am not ashamed of the gospel of Christ, for it is the power of God to salvation for everyone who *believes*, for the Jew first and also for the Greek. For in it the righteousness of God is revealed from *faith* to *faith*; as it is written, 'The just shall live by *faith*'" (Romans 1:16, 17). To the Ephesians, Paul wrote: "For by grace you have been saved through *faith*, and that not of yourselves; it is the gift of God, not of works, lest anyone should boast" Ephesians 2:8, 9). In both letters, Paul stresses the importance of *faith* or *believing*. Jesus Himself said that our "work" is to "*believe* in Him whom He [God the Father] sent" (John 6:29; all emphasis mine).

What does it mean to believe the "gospel of Christ"? Simply put, it is believing that Jesus, the Lamb of God, died in our place (1 Peter 2:24). He paid the death penalty for us. Not only that. He lived a perfect life of righteousness and credits it to our account! (Romans 4:5). Wait, there's more. He rose from the dead and is now our High Priest in Heaven and is interceding for us (Romans 8:34). He is "able to save to the uttermost those who come to God through Him" (Hebrews 7:25). That is the "gospel of Christ," which is the "science of salvation."

Paul said that the gospel is for *everyone* who believes. Everyone could be saved, but not everyone *chooses* to believe the gospel. Believing is vital. When Abraham (then Abram) was advanced in years and Sarah was passed child-bearing age, "God took him outside at night and said, 'Look now toward heaven, and count the stars if you are able to number them.' And He said to him, 'So shall your descendents be.' And he *believed* in the Lord, and He *accounted* it to him for righteousness" (emphasis mine). When we believe that Jesus died for us and lived a perfect life for us, it is credited as righteousness to our account.

God desires our love with a desire stronger than death. Our Father God has given everything that He possibly could to save us. He has given us His only Son to be one of us, a human being, *forever* ! Actions do speak louder than words. What more could God do? Love cannot be forced; only love can bring forth love. In the words of Ellen White:

> Jesus did not come to men with commands and threatenings, but with love that is without a parallel. Love begets love; and thus the love of Christ displayed upon the cross woos and wins the sinner, and binds him, repenting, to the cross, believing and adoring the matchless depths of a Savior's love. Christ came to the world to perfect a righteous character for many, and to elevate the fallen race. But only a few of the millions in our world will accept the righteousness and excellency of his character, and fulfill the requirements given to secure their happiness.[1]

What are God's requirements to secure our happiness? How do we fulfill them? Ellen White answers this question in the book Christ's Object Lessons:[2]

> All His gifts are to be used in blessing humanity, in relieving the suffering and the needy. We are to feed the hungry, to

clothe the naked, to care for the widow and the fatherless, to minister to the distressed and downtrodden. God never meant that the widespread misery in the world should exist. He never meant that one man should have an abundance of the luxuries of life, while the children of others should cry for bread. The means over and above the actual necessities of life are entrusted to man to do good, to bless humanity. The Lord says, "Sell that ye have, and give alms." Luke 12:33. Be "ready to distribute, willing to communicate." 1 Tim. 6:18. "When thou makest a feast, call the poor, the maimed, the lame, the blind." Luke 14:13. "Loose the bands of wickedness," "undo the heavy burdens," "let the oppressed go free," "break every yoke." "Deal thy bread to the hungry," "bring the poor that are cast out to thy house." "When thou seest the naked, . . . cover him." "Satisfy the afflicted soul." Isa. 58:6, 7, 10. "Go ye into all the world, and preach the gospel to every creature." Mark 16:15. These are the Lord's commands. Are the great body of professed Christians doing this work?

When we accept Jesus as our Savior, we also accept Him as our Lord. We are to make an entire, unreserved surrender of our will. We were bought at a price, the precious blood of Jesus. We no longer live for the things of this world. We live to carry out the plan God has for our lives. He has things for us to do! (Ephesians 2:10).

We are to have a part in the Great Commission that Jesus gave His church: making disciples, baptizing them, and teaching them (Matthew 28:19, 20). We are to use the talent(s) He has given us to advance His kingdom (Matthew 25:14–30). We are to bear the fruit of the Holy Spirit: "love, joy, peace, longsuffering, kindness, goodness, faithfulness, gentleness, and self-control" (Galatians 5:22, 23). We are to cooperate with the Holy Spirit as He transforms us from being self-centered to being other-centered.

Believing that Jesus has credited His perfect righteousness to our account is paramount, but is that all there is to it? The apostle James answers that question with a resounding: "Faith without works is dead"

(James 2:20).

From the pen of Ellen White, we read:

> It is not a conclusive evidence that a man is a Christian because he manifests spiritual ecstasy under extraordinary circumstances. Holiness is not rapture: it is an entire surrender of the will to God; it is living by every word that proceeds from the mouth of God; it is doing the will of our Heavenly Father; it is trusting God in trial, in darkness as well as in the light; it is walking by faith and not by sight; it is relying on God with unquestioning confidence, and resting in His love.[3]

Our High Calling

We have a high calling—to be like Jesus! To give glory to God (i.e., to reflect His character) is part of the first angel's message of Revelation 14. Before anyone gets discouraged about meeting this high calling, let's look at what Paul wrote to the Philippians. Right after telling them to "work out your own salvation with fear and trembling" he told them, "for it is *God who works in you* both to will and to do for His good pleasure" (Philippians 2:12, 13, emphasis mine).

It is God who says, "'This is the covenant that I will make with them after those days, says the LORD: *I will* put My laws into their hearts, and in their minds *I will* write them,' then He adds, 'Their sins and their lawless deeds I will remember no more'" (Hebrews 10:16, 17, emphasis mine).

Our goal is to be like Jesus, but our salvation is not based on how close we come to that goal. Our salvation is based on the perfect life of Jesus! May we rest in that wonderful knowledge on Sabbath and have the true understanding of what it means to rest—not depending upon our own works for salvation, but resting wholly on what Jesus *has already accomplished* for us! And may God's Holy Spirit give us the wisdom to be able to present that good news to others in a winsome way.

I am a long way from God's high calling of what He wants me to be, but I know that by the power of God's grace and the power of the Holy

Spirit, He has brought me a long way from where I started. I am thankful for God's patience and His willingness to forgive (1 John 1:9). I am thankful for the untiring work of the Third Person of the Godhead, the Holy Spirit.

God's Work in Us

I am confident that God is able to finish the work He has begun in me and He can finish His work in you too. I thank the apostle Paul for his encouraging words to the Philippians that we can apply to ourselves as well: "being confident of this very thing, that *He who has begun a good work in you will complete it* until the day of Jesus Christ" (Philippians 1:6). Remember, it is *His* work! As He said to Moses, "Speak also to the children of Israel, saying: 'Surely My Sabbaths you shall keep, for it is a sign between Me and you throughout your generations, that you may know that *I am the LORD who sanctifies you* (Exodus 31:13, emphasis mine). *He is Almighty God, and nothing is too hard for Him!* (Jeremiah 32:27).

I am so thankful for the Holy Bible that has given me a clear picture of the true meaning of life on planet earth. I now understand how life on earth started, how this planet was hijacked by an angel gone bad, and why there is suffering and death in this world. God gave His own Son to die for me. I have no doubt that He loves me exceedingly. And that goes for you too!

The New Earth

I get excited thinking about the New Earth, the beautiful meadows, forests, lakes, and streams—even without fishing! He has promised me something better than a four-pound brook trout! Better than all of that, we will see God and talk to Him face to face! I have a hard time grasping that, but the Bible says it and I believe it.

I am so glad to know that throughout the eons of time, the entire universe will be safe. "Affliction will not rise up a second time!" (Nahum 1:9). Praise be to God the Father, Jesus Christ the Son, and God the Holy Spirit!

1. White, E. G. 1875. Review and Herald, March 4, 1875.

2. White, E. G. 1941. *Christ's Object Lessons*. Review and Herald Publishing Association, Washington, DC, 370, 371.

3. White, E. G. 1911. *The Acts of the Apostles*, Pacific Press Publishing Association, Mountain View, California, 51.

Chapter 31
Epilogue, Recommendations, and Resources

A wise man will hear and increase learning, and a man of understanding will attain wise counsel. - Proverbs 1:5

I hope this book has been a blessing to you. May you be blessed knowing that our Father God and Jesus love you and that They want to live with you forever on a beautiful New Earth.

If you have not yet accepted Jesus as your personal Savior, now is the time! "Behold, now is the accepted time; behold, now is the day of salvation" (2 Corinthians 6:2). "Behold, I stand at the door and knock. If anyone hears My voice and opens the door, I will come in to him and dine with him, and he with Me" (Revelation 3:20).

If you accepted Jesus before but have drifted away from a relationship with Him, now is the time to recommit your life to Him. Do not put it off. You do not know if you will be alive tomorrow.

On February 3, 2019, four people inside a California home were watching the Super Bowl game when a plane crashed through the roof, killing them all. As they watched the game, little did they know that their lives would soon come to an end.

Growing in a Relationship with God

The Bible is the best way to hear God speaking to you. If you are new at it, begin with the Gospels, especially the book of John. After you are familiar with the Gospels and other books of the New Testament, start reading the Old Testament beginning in Genesis.

Before you start reading the Bible, ask God for His Holy Spirit to give you understanding. As you read, you can talk to God. If there is something you do not understand, ask Him for help. You may not receive an immediate answer, but often it will come later. Do not let Bible verses you do not understand bother you.

To keep advancing, put into practice what you understand! Do not wait until you understand everything. Expect to be always learning. Even on the New Earth, we will continue learning. Study the Bible with others. We learn from each other, and as we meet together, we draw closer to one another. Believers in Christ are all brothers and sisters in the family of God.

Start each day with prayer. Surrender your will to God and invite the Holy Spirit to take charge of your life. Claim the promises God has given us in the Bible.

Have a forgiving heart toward anyone who has hurt you. Pray for him or her. I have made it a practice to pray that people who have hurt me will be my neighbor on the New Earth. I know that all those living on the New Earth will be restored in God's image and will make good neighbors. I also recognize that God is not done restoring me; my character still needs work. We all need God's grace and mercy!

For More Spiritual Growth

God has given extra help to those living in the time of the end. Based on my extensive research, I am totally convinced that Ellen White was God's messenger and prophet. I have been tremendously blessed by reading her books. If you have any bias about her, I ask you to put it away and examine her life and writings for yourself. Expect to see and hear negative comments about her. Would you expect the devil not to disparage a true prophet of God? Throughout history, Satan has disparaged all of God's prophets. Think how successful he was in vilifying the world's greatest Prophet. He was so successful that the very people who were looking for Him crucified Him!

If you have not yet accepted Jesus as your Savior, I recommend reading *Steps to Christ*,[1] followed by *The Desire of Ages*,[2] and *Christ's*

Object Lessons.[3] If you are already a Christian, you will love Jesus even more after reading these books. To better understand the Old Testament, read *Patriarchs and Prophets*[4] and *Prophets and Kings*.[5]

I highly recommend that everyone read *The Great Controversy*.[6] This book is a history of the Christian church. The first half looks backward in time. It begins with the destruction of Jerusalem, a faint shadow of the destruction of the world that will occur prior to the return of Jesus. It covers the persecution of the early Christians and the assimilation of pagan customs and Greek philosophy into the teachings of the church. It covers the reformation of the church by God's light bearers: the Waldenses, John Wycliffe, Huss and Jerome, Martin Luther and Zwingli, Cranmer, Latimer, Knox, the Huguenots, John and Charles Wesley, and William Miller.

The remainder of the book, based on Bible prophecy, takes us into the future. Future events prophesied in the books of Daniel and Revelation are made plain. You will see the major role that the United States will play in end time events. You will see how the Sabbath of the Fourth Commandment becomes the line in the sand to divide those who are loyal to God and those who are following the devil. Finally, the book ends with the devil meeting his end and God's people receiving their reward. I love reading the last chapter and will quote the last paragraph:

> The great controversy is ended. Sin and sinners are no more. The entire universe is clean. One pulse of harmony and gladness beats through the vast creation. From Him who created all, flow life and light and gladness, throughout the realms of illimitable space. From the minutest atom to the greatest world, all things, animate and inanimate, in their unshadowed beauty and perfect joy, declare that God is love.

I am praying that you will read *The Great Controversy* so that you will be well prepared as the final events described in Revelation unfold. But just in case you do not, I will follow the example of Jesus who said, "And now I have told you before it comes, that when it does come to pass, you may believe" (John 14:29).

I will tell you something that is going to happen that you would never think possible in this land of the free and home of the brave. One day, despite the Constitution guaranteeing us freedom of religion, the United States will pass a law to enforce Sunday worship. Then everyone will have to choose between obeying the law of the land or the law of God. History will repeat itself. What happened in Daniel's time— choosing between the law of the land and the law of God— will happen in our time. Read about what happened to Daniel and his three friends in chapters 3 and 6 of the book of Daniel.

Future events are easily understood in *The Great Controversy*, but I also recommend that you see it in the Bible. Study the books of Daniel and Revelation. I highly recommend the Truth Link Bible studies to guide you. You can obtain a set from Light Bearers Ministry (https://www.lightbearers.org/resources/).

Other good Bible studies are available at these web sites:

- Secrets Unsealed, https://secretsunsealed.org/
- Amazing Facts, https://www.amazingfacts.org/
- It Is Written, https://www.itiswritten.com/
- Voice of Prophecy, https://www.voiceofprophecy.com/
- White Horse Media, https://www.whitehorsemedia.com/
- Jesus 101, http://jesus101.tv/

Here are two websites with Bible study tools that I use a lot:

- Bible Gateway, https://www.biblegateway.com/
- Blue Letter Bible, https://www.blueletterbible.org/search.cfm

For some good science websites, try:

- Creation Study Center, http://creationstudycenter.com/resources/videos/
- Creation-Evolution Headlines, https://crev.info/

- Geoscience Research Institute, https://www.grisda.org/
- Institute for Creation Research, https://www.icr.org
- Discovery Institute, https://www.discovery.org/
- The John 10:10 Project
https://thejohn1010project.com/

An excellent video depicting the most recent events of the Reformation, the Great Religious Awakening of the 1800s, and the parts played by William Miller and Ellen White may be seen here:

- Tell the World, https://telltheworld.adventist.org/

For a true story about a preacher who, after researching the subject of hell, came to the conclusion that God does not burn people forever, watch *Hell and Mr. Fudge.*

- http://www.hellandmrfudge.org/

For inspiring music and sermons, listen to:

- KROH – Radio of Hope, 91.1 FM or https://www radioofhope.org

For Some Good Health Resources

- Learn more about the eight principles for a healthy life style: http://newstart.com/

- Join Dr. David DeRose, MD, MPH for *30 days to Natural Diabetes and High Blood Pressure Control*: https://www.compasshealth.net/help-for-high-blood-pressure/.

- If you want hands-on experience with plant-based cooking and live in the Port Townsend or Sequim, Washington area, try one of Heather Reseck's cooking classes. If you do not live near these areas, Heather offers plant-based recipes and resources online. She is a registered dietitian nutritionist specializing in plant-based cooking and nutrition. For more information: https://www.heatherreseck.com/

- If you would like to learn natural strategies to prevent and reverse chronic diseases including heart disease and diabetes, view Dr. David DeRose's Life Start Seminars: https://lifestartseminars.com

One Final Thought

Understanding the books of Daniel and Revelation is important. That is why God gave us these books. But to be saved and meet Jesus when He returns, understanding the prophecies is not enough. To be saved, you need to know Jesus as your Savior and Lord (John 17:3). It is my prayer that you will choose a relationship with Jesus and grow daily in that relationship.

1. White, E. G. Not dated. *Steps to Christ.* Pacific Press Publishing Association, Nampa, Idaho.

2. White, E. G. 1898. *The Desire of Ages.* Pacific Press Publishing Association, Mountain View, California.

3. White, E. G. 1900. *Christ's Object Lessons.* Review and Herald Publishing Association, Washington, DC.

4. White, E. G. 1958. *Patriarchs and Prophets.* Review and Herald Publishing Association, Mountain View, California.

5. White, E. G. 1917. *Prophets and Kings.* Pacific Press Publishing Association, Mountainview, California.

6. White, E. G. 1911. *The Great Controversy.* Review and Herald Publishing Association, Mountain View, California.

Appendix A
Contaminants in Fish

Mercury

The toxicity of mercury and its effect on the central nervous system was first recognized in Minamata, Japan and was named Minamata disease. In May 1956, four patients were admitted to a hospital with the same severe and baffling symptoms. They suffered from very high fever, convulsions, psychosis, loss of consciousness, coma, and finally death. Soon afterward, 13 other patients from fishing villages near Minamata suffered the same symptoms and also died. Local bird life as well as domestic animals exhibited strange behavior and died. In all, 900 people died and 2,265 people, including babies with birth deformities, were affected. After years of study, the cause was found to be mercury poisoning. A chemical plant was discharging large quantities of mercury into Minamata Bay where fish and shellfish were bioaccumulating the metal and passing it on to fishermen and their families.[1]

What occurred in Minamata where large amounts of mercury were discharged into Minamata Bay is an extreme case and hopefully a poisoning of that magnitude will not happen again. However, more subtle poisonings are apparently happening today within a mother's womb. The developing brain with its 100 billion nerve cells is especially susceptible. That is why fish advisories are especially important for women of childbearing age and children.

Children in the Faroe Islands, born to mothers who consumed mercury-contaminated whale meat were tested at 7 years of age and were found to have neuropsychological dysfunctions in the domains of language, attention, and memory, and to a lesser extent in visuospatial and motor functions.[2]

Inuit children, ages 8–14, from the Arctic Region of Quebec were exposed to mercury in the womb of mothers who consumed whale, fish, seal, and walrus. The children exposed to higher mercury levels were four times as likely to have an IQ score below 80, the clinical cut-off for borderline intellectual disability.[3]

In China, 3-day old newborns from fish-eating mothers were given a Neonatal Behavioral Neurological Assessment to estimate neurobehavioral development. Mothers who consumed more fish had higher cord blood mercury levels. Mercury levels were significantly associated with assessment scores.[4]

Mercury is also associated with cardiovascular disease. In an extensive review, mercury toxicity was found to be highly correlated with high blood pressure, coronary heart disease, heart attack, and stroke. The researchers believed that the protective effect of omega-3 fatty acids was diminished by the occurrence of mercury.[5]

PCBs

PCBs first received notoriety in 1968 when a leaking heat exchanger contaminated rice oil in Kyushu, Japan. Major symptoms of the 2000 people poisoned were dermal and ocular lesions. Other symptoms included irregular menstrual cycles and altered immune response.[6] Symptoms relating to endocrine disruption were discussed in Chapter 16.

In 1979, a similar event occurred in Taiwan when a leaking heat exchanger contaminated rice oil with PCBs. By 1983, there were 2,061 recorded cases of PCB poisoning including 39 babies born from PCB-contaminated mothers. The disease was given the name *yucheng* or oil disease because it came from using rice oil. Acne-like skin eruptions was the most common symptom; other symptoms included follicular accentuations, pigmentation of the skin and nails, and hypersecretion of the Meibomian gland, which contributes oil to tears. Between 1979 and 1983, twenty-four people died from PCB poisoning. Almost half of them died from liver cancer, liver cirrhosis or liver diseases associated with an enlarged liver. Infants born to PCB-poisoned mothers were shorter and weighed less than controls. Eight of the babies died from pneumonia, bronchitis, sepsis (bacterial infection of the blood), and premature and congenital weakness.[7, 8] Children of PCB-contaminated mothers had a higher risk of hearing loss at low frequencies in their right ear.[9]

PCBs were first identified in fish from Lake Michigan in 1968, and since then, have been intensely investigated there.[10] In one study, children of mothers who ate fish were compared to mothers who ate no fish. Newborns of the fish-eating mothers were smaller, had abnormally weak reflexes, reduced responsiveness, reduced motor coordination, and reduced muscle tone. PCB levels in the mother's blood and milk correlated to the amount of fish consumed; levels in the umbilical cord blood correlated to the level in the mother's blood.[11, 12] At 7 months, the children from the fish-eating mothers exhibited decreased visual recognition ability and had possible neurological impairment.[13] At 4 years, they had slower reactions to visual stimuli, more errors and longer times to solve memory tests, diminished attention control and information retention, and possible hyperactivity.[14]

At 11 years, the children were given a battery of IQ and achievement tests, which assessed their reading and arithmetic skills. Test results were correlated with PCB levels in umbilical cord blood and maternal blood and milk. The strongest effects were related to memory and attention. The most highly PCB-exposed children were three times as likely to have low average IQ scores and twice as likely to be at least two years behind in reading comprehension. Although larger quantities of PCBs were transferred in breast-feeding than in utero, there were deficits only in association with transplacental exposure, suggesting that the developing fetal brain is particularly sensitive. It is also notable that PCB levels in the mother's blood and milk at delivery were only slightly higher than in the general population.[15]

About 10 years later, another PCB study was conducted on children from the city of Oswego, located on the shore of Lake Ontario in New York State. Results were remarkably similar to those of the Michigan study. Both studies found that prenatal PCB exposure was associated with lower Full Scale IQ, and both found that Verbal IQ, but not

Performance IQ, was primarily predictive of the IQ deficit. Both studies noted that the Freedom from Distractibility scale scores were significantly poorer in the PCB-exposed children. In the Oswego study, there was an approximate three-point drop in IQ for every 1 nanogram of PCBs per gram of placental tissue. This translated to a six- to seven-point drop in Full Scale IQ and about a nine-point drop in Verbal IQ from the least to the most PCB-exposed groups.[16]

The Wisconsin Department of Health Services and Natural Resources studied a group of older male anglers (median age 60.5 years). For every PCB congener analyzed, blood PCB levels were related to the amount of fish consumed from the Great Lakes as well as from other Wisconsin waterbodies.[17]

In a study of Inuit women and their babies living on the Hudson Bay in northern Quebec, different cognitive disabilities were associated with PCBs, mercury, and lead levels in umbilical cord blood. The infants were tested at 6.5 months and 11 months. PCBs were associated with impairment of visual recognition memory; methylmercury with working memory and an early precursor of executive function; and lead with processing speed.[18]

PCBs in mother's blood have been linked to autism. In a study of Southern California children, Autism Spectrum Disorder (ASD) risk was elevated for a number of PCB congeners and one PCB congener was associated with higher risk for Intellectual Disability (ID).[19]

In a study of over 69,000 Swedish men and women, PCBs were found to counteract the beneficial aspects of omega-3 fatty acids in preventing heart disease.[20]

1. Juan, S. 2006. *The Minamata disaster—50 years on Lessons learned?* The Register 14 July 2006. https://www.theregister.co.uk/2006/07/14/the_odd_body_minimata_disaster/

2. Grandjean, P., P. Weihe, R. F. White, F. Debes, S. Araki, K. Yokoyama, K. Murata, N. Sorensen, R. Dahl, and P. J. Jorgensen. 1997. Cognitive deficit in 7-year-old children with prenatal exposure to methylmercury. *Neurotoxicology Teratology* 19(6):417–428.

3. Jacobson, J. L., G. Muckle, P. Ayotte, E. Dewailly, S. W. Jacobson. 2015. Relation of prenatal methylmercury exposure from environmental sources to childhood IQ. *Environmental Health Perspectives* 123(8):827–833.

4. Wu, J., T. Ying, Z. Shen, and H. Wang. 2014. Effect of low-level prenatal mercury exposure on neonate neurobehavioral development in China. *Pediatric Neurology* 51:93–99.

5.Houston, M. C. 2014. The role of mercury in cardiovascular disease. *Journal of Cardiovascular Diseases & Diagnosis.* 2(5):1–8.

6.Yasunobu, A. 2001. Polychlorinated Biphenyls, Polychloronated Dibenzo-*p*-dioxins, and Polychlorinated Dibenzofurans as Endocrine Disrupters—What We Have Learned from Yusho Disease. *Environmental Research* 86 (1):2–11.

7. Hsu, S. T., C. I. Ma, S. K. H. Hsu, S. S. Wu, N. H. M. HSU, C. C. Yeh, and S. B. Wu. 1985. Discovery and Epidemiology of PCB Poisoning in Taiwan: A Four-Year Followup. *Environmental Health Perspectives* 59:5–10.

https://ehp.niehs.nih.gov/cms/attachment/da0a0be8-39e4-41e2-9dd9-c8bd3f089a0c/ehp.59-1568088.pdf

8. Rogan, W. J., B. C. Gladen, K. L. Hung, S. L. Koong, L. Y. Shih, J. S. Taylor, Y. C. Wu, D. Yang, N. B. Ragon, and C. C. Hsu. 1988. Congenital Poisoning by Polychlorinated Biphenyls and Their Contaminants in Taiwan. *Science* 241:334–336.

https://pdfs.semanticscholar.org/0dc1/c74d7ce9db84ae38214d1a95e416dfa5b730.pdf

9. Li, M. C., H. P. Wu, C. Y. Yang, P. C. Chen, G. H. Lambert, and Y. L. Guo. 2015. Gestational exposure to polychlorinated biphenyls and dibenzo furans induced asymmetric hearing loss: Yucheng children. *Environmental research* 137:65–71.

10. Hornbuckle, K. C., D. L. Carlson, D. L. Swackhamer, J. E. Baker, and S. J. Eisenreich 2006. *Polychlorinated biphenyls in the Great Lakes.* The Handbook of Environmental Chemistry, Volume 5. Part N:13–70; Springer-Verlag Berlin, Heidelberg (Published online 20 December 2005).

11. Jacobson, J., S. Jacobson, G. Fein, P. Swartz, and J. Dowler. 1984. Prenatal exposure to an environmental toxin: A test of the multiple effects model. *Developmental Psychology* 20 (4): 523–532.

12. Fein, G. G., J. L. Jacobson, S. W. Jacobson, P. M. Swartz, and J. K. Dowler. 1984. Prenatal exposure to polychlorinated biphenyls: effects on birth size and gestational age. *Journal of Pediatrics* 105:315–320.

13. Jacobson, S. W., G. G. Fein, J. L. Jacobson, P. M. Swartz, and J. K. Dowler. 1985. The effects of PCB exposure on visual recognition memory. *Child Development* 56:853–860.

14. Jacobson, J. L., S. W. Jacobson, and H. E. B. Humphrey. 1990. Effects of in utero exposure to polychlorinated biphenyls and related contaminants on cognitive functioning in young children. *Journal of Pediatrics* 116:38–45.

15. Jacobson, J. L., and S. W. Jacobson. 1996. Intellectual impairment in children exposed to polychlorinated biphenyls in utero. *New England Journal of Medicine* 335 (11):783–9.

16. Stewart, P. W., E. Lonky. J. Reihman, J. Pagano, B. B. Gump, and T. Darvill. 2008. The relationship between prenatal PCB exposure and intelligence (IQ) in 9-year-old children. *Environmental Health Perspectives* 116(10):1416–1422.

17. Christensen, K. Y., B. A. Thompson, M. Werner, K. Malecki, P. Imm, and H. A. Anderson. 2016. Levels of persistent contaminants in relation to fish consumption among older male anglers in Wisconsin. *International Journal of Hygiene and Health* 219(2):184–194.

18. O. Boucher, G. Muckle, J. L. Jacobson, R. C. Carter, M. Kaplan-Estrin, P. Ayotte, E. Dewailly, and S. W. Jacobson. 2014. Domain-Specific effects of prenatal exposure to PCBs, mercury, and lead on infant cognition: results from the environmental contaminants and child development study in Nunavik. *Environmental Health Perspectives* 122 (3):310–316.

19. Lyall, K., L. A. Croen, A. Sjodin, C. K. Yoshida, O. Zerbo, M. Kharrazi, and G. C. Windam. 2017. Polychlorinated biphenyl and organochlorine pesticide concentrations in maternal mid-pregnancy serum samples: association with Autism Spectrum Disorder and

Intellectual Disability. *Environmental Health Perspectives*, online. https://ehp.niehs.nih.gov/doi/full/10.1289/EHP277

20. Akesson, A, C. Donat-Vargas, M. Berglund, A. Glynn, A. Wolk, and M. Kippler. 2019. Dietary exposure to polychlorinated biphenyls and risk of heart failure — a population-based prospective cohort study. *Environment International* 126:1-6.

Appendix B
Prophecies Fulfilled

Rejected by His own people, the Jews

He is despised and rejected by men, a Man of sorrows and acquainted with grief. And we hid, as it were, our faces from Him; He was despised, and we did not esteem Him. Isaiah 53:3

He came to His own, and His own did not receive Him. John 1:11

Sold for thirty pieces of silver

Then I said to them, "If it is agreeable to you, give me my wages; and if not, refrain." So they weighed out for my wages thirty pieces silver. Zechariah 11:12

and said, "What are you willing to give me if I deliver Him to you?" And they counted out to him thirty pieces of silver. Matthew 26:15

Born in Bethlehem

But you, Bethlehem Ephrathah, Though you are Little among the thousands of Judah, Yet out of you shall come forth to Me; The One to be Ruler in Israel, Whose goings forth are from of old, From everlasting. Micah 5:2

Joseph also went up from Galilee, out of the city of Nazareth, into

Judea, to the city of David, which is called Bethlehem, because he was of the house and lineage of David, to be registered with Mary, his betrothed wife, who was with child. Luke 2:4, 5

Born of a virgin

Therefore the Lord Himself will give you a sign: Behold, the virgin shall conceive and bear a Son, and shall call His name Immanuel. Isaiah 7:14

Now in the sixth month the angel Gabriel was sent by God to a city of Galilee named Nazareth, to a virgin betrothed to a man whose name was Joseph, of the house of David. The virgin's name was Mary. Luke 1:26, 27

Betrayed by a friend

Even my own familiar friend in whom I trusted, who ate my bread, has lifted up his heel against me. Psalm 41:9

And while He was still speaking, behold a multitude; and he who was called Judas, one of the twelve, went before them and drew near to Jesus to kiss Him. But Jesus said to him, "Judas, are you betraying the Son of Man with a kiss?" Luke 22:47, 48

Spat upon and smitten

I gave My back to those who struck Me, and My cheeks to those who plucked out the beard;
I did not hide My face from shame and spitting. Isaiah 50:6

Then they spat in His face and beat Him; and struck Him with palms of their hands, saying, "Prophesy to us, Christ! Who is the one who struck You?" Matthew 26:67

Scorned and mocked

All those who see Me ridicule Me; they shoot out the lip, they shake the head, saying, "He trusted in the LORD, let Him rescue Him; let Him deliver Him, since He delights in Him!" Psalm 22:7, 8

And people stood looking on. But even the rulers with them sneered, saying, "He saved others; let Him save Himself if He is the Christ, the chosen of God." Luke 23:35

Appendix C
In the Spirit and Power of Elias

The following excerpts are taken from the chapter *In the Spirit and Power of Elias* in the book *Prophets and Kings* by Ellen White.[1]

Before entering the Promised Land, the Israelites were admonished by Moses to "keep the Sabbath day to sanctify it." Deuteronomy 5:12. The Lord designed that by a faithful observance of the Sabbath command, Israel should continually be reminded of their accountability to Him as their Creator and their Redeemer. While they should keep the Sabbath in the proper spirit, idolatry could not exist; but should the claims of this precept of the Decalogue be set aside as no longer binding, the Creator would be forgotten and men would worship other gods. "I gave them My Sabbaths," God declared, "to be a sign between Me and them, that they might know that I am the Lord that sanctify them." Yet "they despised My judgments, and walked not in My statutes, but polluted My Sabbaths: for their heart went after their idols." And in His appeal to them to return to Him, He called their attention anew to the importance of keeping the Sabbath holy. "I am the Lord your God," He said; "walk in My statutes, and keep My judgments, and do them; and hallow My Sabbaths; and they shall be a sign between Me and you, that ye may know that I am the Lord your God." Ezekiel 20:12, 16, 19, 20.

In calling the attention of Judah to the sins that finally brought upon them the Babylonian Captivity, the Lord declared: "Thou hast . . . profaned My Sabbaths." "Therefore have I poured out Mine indignation upon them; I have consumed them with the fire of My wrath: their own way have I recompensed upon their heads." Ezekiel 22:8, 31.

At the restoration of Jerusalem, in the days of Nehemiah, Sabbathbreaking was met with the stern inquiry, "Did not your fathers thus, and did not our God bring all this evil upon us, and upon this city? yet ye bring more wrath upon Israel by profaning the Sabbath." Nehemiah 13:18.

Christ, during His earthly ministry, emphasized the binding claims of the Sabbath; in all His teaching He showed reverence for the institution He Himself had given. In His days the Sabbath had become so perverted that its observance reflected the character of selfish and arbitrary men rather than the character of God. Christ set aside the false teaching by which those who claimed to know God had misrepresented Him. Although followed with merciless hostility by the rabbis, He did not even appear to conform to their requirements, but went straight forward keeping the Sabbath according to the law of God.

In unmistakable language He testified to His regard for the law of Jehovah. "Think not that I am come to destroy the law, or the prophets," He said; "I am not come to destroy, but to fulfill. For verily I say unto you, Till heaven and earth pass, one jot or one tittle shall in no wise pass from the law, till all be fulfilled. Whosoever therefore shall break one of these least commandments, and shall teach men so, he shall be called the least in the kingdom of heaven: but whosoever shall do and teach them, the same shall be called great in the kingdom of heaven." Matthew 5:17-19.

During the Christian dispensation, the great enemy of man's happiness has made the Sabbath of the fourth commandment an object of special attack. Satan says, "I will work at cross purposes with God. I will empower my followers to set aside God's memorial, the seventh-day Sabbath. Thus I will show the world that the day sanctified and blessed by God has been changed. That day shall not live in the minds of the people. I will obliterate the memory of it. I will place in its stead a day that does not bear the credentials of God, a day that cannot be a sign between God and His people. I will lead those who accept this day to place upon it the sanctity that God placed upon the seventh day.

"Through my vicegerent, I will exalt myself. The first day will be extolled, and the Protestant world will receive this spurious sabbath as genuine. Through the nonobservance of the Sabbath that God instituted, I will bring His law into contempt. The words, 'A sign between Me and you throughout your generations,' I will make to serve on the side of my sabbath.

"Thus the world will become mine. I will be the ruler of the earth, the prince of the world. I will so control the minds under my power that God's Sabbath shall be a special object of contempt. A sign? I will make the observance of the seventh day a sign of disloyalty to the authorities of earth. Human laws will be made so stringent that men and women will not dare to observe the seventh-day Sabbath. For fear of wanting food and clothing, they will join with the world in transgressing God's law. The earth will be wholly under my dominion."

Through the setting up of a false sabbath, the enemy thought to change times and laws. But has he really succeeded in changing God's law? The words of the thirty-first chapter of Exodus are the answer. He who is the same yesterday, today, and forever, has declared of the seventh-day Sabbath: "It is a sign between Me and you throughout your generations." "It is a sign . . . forever." Exodus 31:13, 17. The changed signpost is pointing the wrong way, but God has not changed. He is still the mighty God of Israel. "Behold, the nations are as a drop of a bucket, and are counted as the small dust of the balance: behold, He taketh up the isles as a very little thing. And Lebanon is not sufficient to burn, nor the beasts thereof sufficient for a burnt offering. All nations before Him are as nothing; and they are counted to Him less than nothing, and vanity." Isaiah 40:15-17. And He is just as jealous for His law now as He was in the days of Ahab and Elijah.

But how is that law disregarded! Behold the world today in open rebellion against God. This is in truth a froward generation, filled with ingratitude, formalism, insincerity, pride, and apostasy. Men neglect the Bible and hate truth. Jesus sees His law rejected, His love despised, His ambassadors treated with indifference. He has spoken by His mercies, but these have been unacknowledged; He has spoken by warnings, but these have been unheeded. The temple courts of the human soul have been turned into places of unholy traffic. Selfishness, envy, pride, malice—all are cherished.

Many do not hesitate to sneer at the word of God. Those who believe that word just as it reads are held up to ridicule. There is a growing contempt for law and order, directly traceable to a violation of the plain commands of Jehovah. Violence and crime are the result of turning aside from the path of obedience. Behold the wretchedness and misery of multitudes who worship at the shrine of idols and who seek in vain for happiness and peace.

Behold the well-nigh universal disregard of the Sabbath commandment. Behold also the daring impiety of those who, while enacting laws to safeguard the supposed sanctity of the first day of the week, at the same time are making laws legalizing the liquor traffic. Wise above that which is written, they attempt to coerce the consciences of men, while lending their sanction to an evil that brutalizes and destroys the beings created in the image of God. It is Satan himself who inspires such legislation. He well knows that the curse of God will rest on those who exalt human enactments above the divine, and he does all in his power to lead men into the broad road that ends in destruction.

So long have men worshiped human opinions and human

institutions that almost the whole world is following after idols. And he who has endeavored to change God's law is using every deceptive artifice to induce men and women to array themselves against God and against the sign by which the righteous are known. But the Lord will not always suffer His law to be broken and despised with impunity. There is a time coming when "the lofty looks of man shall be humbled, and the haughtiness of men shall be bowed down, and the Lord alone shall be exalted in that day." Isaiah 2:11. Skepticism may treat the claims of God's law with jest, scoffing, and denial. The spirit of worldliness may contaminate the many and control the few, the cause of God may hold its ground only by great exertion and continual sacrifice, yet in the end the truth will triumph gloriously.

In the closing work of God in the earth, the standard of His law will be again exalted. False religion may prevail, iniquity may abound, the love of many may wax cold, the cross of Calvary may be lost sight of, and darkness, like the pall of death, may spread over the world; the whole force of the popular current may be turned against the truth; plot after plot may be formed to overthrow the people of God; but in the hour of greatest peril the God of Elijah will raise up human instrumentalities to bear a message that will not be silenced. In the populous cities of the land, and in the places where men have gone to the greatest lengths in speaking against the Most High, the voice of stern rebuke will be heard. Boldly will men of God's appointment denounce the union of the church with the world. Earnestly will they call upon men and women to turn from the observance of a man-made institution to the observance of the true Sabbath. "Fear God, and give glory to Him," they will proclaim to every nation; "for the hour of His judgment is come: and worship Him that made heaven, and earth, and the sea, and the fountains of waters. . . . If any man worship the beast and his image, and receive his mark in his forehead, or in his hand, the same shall drink of the wine of the wrath of God, which is poured out without mixture into the cup of His indignation." Revelation 14:7-10.

God will not break His covenant, nor alter the thing that has gone out of His lips. His word will stand fast forever as unalterable as His throne. At the judgment this covenant will be brought forth, plainly written with the finger of God, and the world will be arraigned before the bar of Infinite Justice to receive sentence.

Today, as in the days of Elijah, the line of demarcation between God's commandment-keeping people and the worshipers of false gods is clearly drawn. "How long halt ye between two opinions?" Elijah cried; "if the Lord be God, follow Him: but if Baal, then follow him." 1 Kings 18:21. And the message for today is: "Babylon the great is fallen, is fallen. . . . Come out of her, My people, that ye be not partakers of her sins, and that ye receive not of her plagues. For her sins have reached unto heaven, and God hath remembered her iniquities." Revelation 18:2, 4, 5.

The time is not far distant when the test will come to every soul. The observance of the false sabbath will be urged upon us. The contest will be between the commandments of God and the commandments of men. Those who have yielded step by step to worldly demands and conformed to worldly customs will then yield to the powers that be, rather than subject themselves to derision, insult, threatened imprisonment, and death. At that time the gold will be separated from the dross. True godliness will be clearly distinguished from the appearance and tinsel of it. Many a star that we have admired for its brilliance will then go out in darkness. Those who have assumed the ornaments of the sanctuary, but are not clothed with Christ's righteousness, will then appear in the shame of their own nakedness.

Among earth's inhabitants, scattered in every land, there are those who have not bowed the knee to Baal. Like the stars of heaven, which appear only at night, these faithful ones will shine forth when darkness covers the earth and gross darkness the people. In heathen Africa, in the Catholic lands of Europe and of South America, in China, in India, in the islands of the sea, and in all the dark corners of the earth, God has in reserve a firmament of chosen ones that will yet shine forth amidst the darkness, revealing clearly to an apostate world the transforming power of obedience to His law. Even now they are appearing in every nation, among every tongue and people; and in the hour of deepest apostasy, when Satan's supreme effort is made to cause "all, both small and great, rich and poor, free and bond," to receive, under penalty of death, the sign of allegiance to a false rest day, these faithful ones, "blameless and harmless, the sons of God, without rebuke," will "shine as lights in the world." Revelation 13:16; Philippians 2:15. The darker the night, the more brilliantly will they shine.

What strange work Elijah would have done in numbering Israel at the time when God's judgments were falling upon the backsliding people! He could count only one on the Lord's side. But when he said, "I, even I only, am left; and they seek my life," the word of the Lord surprised him, "Yet I have left Me seven thousand in Israel, all the knees which have not bowed unto Baal." 1 Kings 19:14, 18.

Then let no man attempt to number Israel today, but let everyone have a heart of flesh, a heart of tender sympathy, a heart that, like the heart of Christ, reaches out for the salvation of a lost world.

1. White, E. G. 1917. *Prophets and Kings*. Pacific Press Publishing Association, Mountainview, California, 181–189.

Made in the USA
Middletown, DE
11 July 2021